Dedication

To my dad, who lost his life at the age of 41. For those short nine years you raised me, you taught me so much. You showed me how to live life without a care in the world. When I think of the holidays, I think of you stopping at a stop sign or railroad crossing only to turn the music up loud and zydeco dance outside of your truck in the middle of the road. That is what I call care-free living! I love to think back to your laugh that lit up a room at all of the parties you would attend, carrying a crown on the rocks alcoholic beverage in your hand. How does a sound light up a room? Only the resonating, contagious laugh you had could do that. And I can never forget the amazing smile that went with your happiness. It shined like no other.

Dad, you showed me how to enjoy the finer things in life and it all started with your large, black, dually Ford F-150 truck that you rode around in style. When we would go shopping and I couldn't decide which sweatshirt I wanted or what new pair of shoes would be my fresh school year kicks, you'd always say, "Just get both." Talk about finer living and never settling when it comes to getting what you want. I am sure that is why my love language is gifts, because, Dad, you spoiled me rotten and I wouldn't have had my childhood any other way. It turned me into the hard worker that I am today. I watched you raise an amazing family and anything we wanted or needed, you provided through your strong work ethic and what I like to call "boss mentality."

While riding with you in your truck, I remember thinking as a child that I would have a personal driver when I got older. Whether you knew it or not, you always kept me dreaming BIG and thinking I could conquer the world if I set my mind to it. Most importantly, you showed me how to love unconditionally, as you did Mom, and how to give your last dollar to someone who needed it. I recall the many favors you would help your employees with. If they had family matters to take care of and they couldn't show up to work, you kindly gave them the day off. If they had vehicle issues, you picked them up without even asking them why. Even though you were technically their boss, you treated your employees as your friends. I have always admired that about you. I hope to be as amazing of a boss and friend as you were and give back, just as you did. I aspire to be a great parent, just as you were to me and my sisters, because you were such a family-oriented man who showed his love to us everyday, regardless of how busy you were. You loved mom by showering her with

I KILLED

My Father's

KILLER

How What You Are Eating Can
Be Killing You Too

By

Katelyn Foxworth

I Killed My Killer Series

Copyright 2020 © by Katelyn Sonnier

casino and dinner dates. You loved her even more through loving Natalyn and me. You have been and always will be the perfect example of love to me.

To my amazing fiancé (at the time I started writing this book), now husband, DePaul. Thank you for always believing in me, even when I didn't have an ounce of belief in myself. With every crazy, ambitious, and new business idea I would mention to you, you'd never discourage me or call me crazy (at least not to my face). 😊 You kept our dream and our vision alive even when I didn't think it was possible. When the electricity was getting shut off and the eviction notices were coming in just as frequently as the bills, you saw the light at the end of the tunnel. You kept hope alive through it all because you believed that we were going to make it. Thank you for pushing me to always be the best version of myself, even when others thought you were trying to "control me." You saw the potential I had in me when those I loved most didn't. I wouldn't be the woman, wife, and mother that I am today if it wasn't for you.

Thank you for being adamant about pursuing me, and our dreams, for pushing both of us to be better versions of ourselves daily. Whenever I have my physically lazy days, or I forget to do something in my business, you hold me accountable to get my goals done while still giving me the perfect amount of grace and love. Much appreciation to you, DePaul, for being the amazing, Godly man I love you for. With all of the insane decisions we make, from big city moves to crazy personal changes in our lifestyle, I know we are protected because of your Godly counsel and walk with Christ.

Most importantly, I thank The Man Himself, God! If it was not for Him, we wouldn't be where we are today and where we are headed tomorrow. He is the reason for our motivation, our inspiration and our daily sanctification! Our gifts are His and I pray we use them to glorify Him. When I wanted to put the pen down and stop writing, He was the one who whispered that I needed to keep going because someone needed to hear my story. Just as a coach and friend of mine, Michelle O'Conner, once mentioned in a story to me that someone is in heaven and died a little too early because I didn't use my gifts.

Table of contents

Introduction

You Are What You Eat

You may have heard the saying before, "You are what you eat." I agree with this saying 100% and I will elaborate more on this throughout this book, explaining how I was a busted can of biscuits (shout-out to my highschool friend, Jessica, for that saying) and transformed into what I like to call a healthier, sexier looking croissant, who could actually fit in her jeans without love handles hanging off the sides.

Turning into what you eat is something I did not know growing up. I had to go through deep depression, obesity, and many other low-blows in life for me to realize that what we put into our bodies eventually becomes who we are. I wish someone would have told me when I was younger that when you put good foods into your body, you get great results. Not only physically, but mentally as well. Verses when you feed your body unhealthy foods, you become well...*unhealthy*!

Growing up, the only thing that mattered to me when I ate was how good the food tasted. I never ordered anything off of the menu because it would make me feel better after I ate it. No. I ordered my food thinking short-term. "What is going to taste good in the next few minutes after the kitchen finishes cooking it?" I would ask myself. "Hmm. Am I in the mood for some fried pork chops and red beans, or do I want to keep it simple with a BLT?" I know that most of us order our meals based off of those same standards: What are we in the mood for? That is exactly how I thought too.

My relationship with food was bad, (I mean *bad*, bad) and it showed on the inside and out. My love for unhealthy food showed physically in how I looked, emotionally in how I felt, and how I treated those around me.

I would wake up and live to eat. You know, when all you can look forward to is that amazing meal you've got planned, so you don't eat anything all morning until that most anticipated meal is ready, and then you overindulge in it. Especially on the holidays! That is when I would keep eating, even when I was full. We've all been there, done that. You know, that moment when your stomach is so full it almost hurts, but you stare at all the entrees you haven't even tried yet and your self-control is shattered. And oh wait, they have dessert?! Well, you just *have* to try that delicious-looking piece of red velvet cake that practically sings your name. Who knows when your next opportunity to try it will be; it may not be until the next holiday season. That was my mindset anyway. I would stuff my face and stomach, even though I could barely take another bite. At this point, I would only be eating because I wanted that taste. All I was looking forward to was that sweet and savory flavor hitting my taste buds in the back of my throat. Those factors shouldn't have mattered to me as much as they did in those moments.

The truth is, who cares when you'll get to have a slice of red velvet cake or your aunt's famous German chocolate cake. I am sure you'll be presented with many more delicious desserts several other times throughout life. When those treats are presented to us, we need to ask ourselves, "Are we in control of what we are eating or just living for the moment?" What we need to keep in mind is that we are supposed to eat to live! You know, eating good foods to help my body grow strong bones and muscles, **not fat!**

Now that I am in my 20s, I try not to judge my food solely on taste as I did all the time growing up. I determine what I eat by how it will make me feel after I eat it. I've come to this conclusion after much trial and error, and I am still a work in progress. Why? Because I am human and sometimes what tastes better at that moment seems like a better decision than the spinach salad. And that is what this book is going to show you; my journey from my lowest of lows as the fat girl without a daddy, to the thriving, vibrant woman I see myself as today and what areas of life this affects.

Determining my food based on how it will make me feel as a human, isn't something that came naturally or easy to me, especially since I was born and raised in the South and we love to eat what we call *soul food*. In Southern Louisiana, when it comes to food, all we care about is:

1. Is it fried?

2. Is it smothered in sauce or does it have a good gravy?

3. Is it seasoned well with some hot sauce, Tony Chachere's seasoning, or maybe even some Season All?

Not once does the question come to mind: How will this make me feel and how will I look after I eat this?

That is why, when I was growing up, you could probably roll me around anywhere you needed to take me. I was an obese child, looking like a chubby-cheeked rolly polly. Since I was a young child, I was short with a protruding belly like several kids who suffer from childhood obesity. The only problem with mine was that I did not grow out of it like many of my peers did as we were going from elementary school to junior high. All of my other friends started to lose their "baby fat" the older they got, yet I was still chunky! I was getting more and more "baby fat" because of my unhealthy daily habits.

As I was getting heavier, I didn't think to realize that maybe it was because of the pack of oreos I was eating when I got off the school bus. And I didn't know it was the compound effect of eating mine and my friend's bread rolls for lunch, even though she didn't want hers anyway. As my stomach started to push the buttons on my shirts further and further out, straining them to the limit, my self esteem sunk lower and lower. That wasn't motivation for me to change my eating habits at all. It only made me want to continue eating and sleeping even more; I couldn't see a way out. I hated the way I looked when I saw myself in a picture with my friends. I despised the reflection staring back at me in the mirror.

I had family members telling me, "You are just big boned, Katelyn, so get used to being bigger because you'll never be like one of those skinny girls." I believed every word, and I was devastated. I began classifying myself as big boned, because it was easier to deal with than calling it what it was. Having family, people we are supposed to get love and support from, tell us we'll never be skinny (which is almost synonymous with beauty, thanks to what the media is shaping young girls' impressions into at this time period) is very hard and depressing.

It was not until I turned 20 that I began to put two and two together. Brace yourselves, this next part may be hard for some of you to hear. I began to realize I couldn't blame anyone else for the life I was choosing to live and the size that I was. The full blame landed squarely on my shoulders alone. I started to realize that it was the foods I was feeding myself that resulted in the body I had to live with. I learned that I was not big boned; that "being big boned" wasn't even a real thing. It was just something people told themselves and others to make us feel better about being stuck in the unhealthy weight that we are.

This is a fact of human nature: we tend to believe what others say about us, especially those we trust most, like friends and family. We grow up our entire lives not even realizing it. I have friends who believe they are shy because their mother called them "shy" growing up. Or maybe you can relate because your parents told you you wouldn't amount to anything. Whatever those terrible lies are, big or small, we have to stop believing what other people have said about us is true! The only way to find out if we are what they say we are is to try it out. When I turned the tables around and began to eat differently, my body revealed to me that I was *not* "big boned and destined to remain that way." Thank you, Lord!

For many of us, we grow up cooking and eating what we have seen our families do for years. Does this necessarily mean that it is the right and healthiest thing to do?

I realized that it could be the foods that my family had grown up eating for generations that determined how long they lived. Was the delicious, savory taste of gumbo and pecan candies year round really worth the detrimental qualities that came with them? If the foods my father ate weren't helping the longevity of his life, could that be what killed him? Come with me on my journey to kill my father's killer, every up and down, twist and turn. Every failure, and every dragging myself back up to keep fighting.

Chapter 1

Happy Halloween

Beep. Beep. Beep. Beep. Beep. Beep. Beep. Beep. Beep. A familiar, yet not so familiar sound. The sound of my father's alarm clock, but it won't stop this time. Usually daddy is quick to turn it off after three beeps, so why won't it stop this morning? I am certain he normally wakes up on time; I know the routine, I've been sleeping in my parents room every night for the first nine years of my life.

"Mom," I slurred out as I sleepily opened my eyes to see what was going on. There mom was, frantically shaking my dad as he lay there beside me, motionless. I was sleeping in my favorite spot, tucked right underneath his arm. The only difference was he didn't feel as warm as he normally does. I heard mom yell, "Mervin! Mervin!

Wake up, Mervin!" But he didn't move. He continued to lay there as stiff as a board.

Man, dad must be sleeping hard this morning, I thought as mom started to call someone. I assumed it was Papa, my grandfather, she was calling. Maybe he had some tips on how to wake up a sleepy bricklayer since Papa was a brick mason himself. Papa and Dad were easy risers who started their work before the roosters were even up.

I was frightened to discover it was not Papa that Mom was calling. I was not prepared for the words I heard her speak next.

"Hello, 911! Yes, I am calling because my husband Mervin won't wake up! I think he's dead!"

After hearing those words come out of my mother's mouth, I did what every little sister would do. I ran across the hallway and into my big sister's room. She had those hippie door beads hanging down across her bedroom door threshold all the way to the floor. I ran across the hallway, busting through those door beads as if they weren't even there, anxious to get to my sister's bedside in a flash and deliver the news to her.

I shouted, "Sissy! Sissy!" I shook her and she finally rolled over. "I think daddy is dead," I told her. Her roll over quickly made its way into a bear hug as she tried to tuck me under the covers with her to put me back to sleep. "It is just a dream," Sissy said. "Go back to sleep, Kay Kay."

I yelled at her, "No! It is not a dream. I was sleeping by daddy then his alarm clock went off and now he won't wake up. Mommy said he is dead."

Then the covers flew off of my older sister as she started running across the hall faster than I'd ever seen her run. Seconds later she was standing over my dad's dead body crying in disbelief. It hit me like a ton of bricks when I saw my sister balling her eyes out as she hugged and squeezed my mom tightly. That is when I realized this was real, from the alarm clock sounding off to my mom calling the police. My father is really dead.

The pain I felt in that moment washed away every joyful memory I had ever experienced in my nine years of living. None of those happy childhood memories mattered to me anymore as I stood over my dad's blue, stone-cold body that I would never see move again. It was then that I felt my body, my emotions, and my life start to go numb as I heard the sirens of the ambulance arriving at our house.

In that moment, my world turned upside down. Could my dad, my best friend, my *everything* really be dead? I had always been a daddy's girl so there was no way my best friend could leave this Earth without me. We still had houses to brick, I had grades to pass, and, eventually of course, I needed my father to walk me down the aisle when prince charming arrived. *He can't be dead*, my nine-year-old self thought.

Being born and raised a practicing Catholic, I call back to those times in the church singing songs like "Do not be afraid, I am with you..." I also remember all of the stories in the Bible where Jesus worked miracles for the sick and dying. If my dad is really dead, then screw the rules because where the hell are you now, God? If you are really here, then why can't you bring my dad back to life? Why would you kill him in his sleep?

Battling these thoughts on God in my head, minutes dragged by like hours. Then my sister grabbed me by my hand and walked me to my room to watch the cartoon *Madeline* until we heard further news on dad's condition. I sat there not even watching the TV, just wondering to myself this has to be a dream. One of those dreams that feel so real, then you wake up and thank God it was not true.

Unfortunately, I never woke up from this nightmare. Moments that felt like lifetimes passed before anyone came into my room to give us an update. Then Mom entered. The update was only that the ambulance had arrived and would be taking my dad, my hero, to the morgue because he was indeed dead.

My younger self still had hope that the paramedics would take out those two electric squares, press it on my dad's chest, and then BOOM! He could come back to life. If that would happen, maybe I would have faith in God again.

What kind of God would take a little girl's father? With no warning. Right out of his sleep, with me sleeping so peacefully in his arms. I was so bitter. I began to hold a giant grudge against God. I felt a hole deep inside of me manifest and I knew that nothing could fill it. That deep, dark hole was now there because God took my dad away from me. That missing piece in my heart was something I knew I would always blame God for and it is the reason I would wake up angry at Him.

The doctors said there was no way to get him back because he had been dead hours before his alarm clock went off. So, they loaded his heavy body onto the stretcher and carried him down the hallway, past my bedroom and out the door to the ambulance.

Still to this day I hate the cartoon *Madeline*. I even hate the movie *Halloween*. It was the last movie we watched together, on the eve of Halloween, curled up just me and my dad and my puppy, Fluffy. Clicking the TV off, his last words to me were, "Come on Skooby. Let's go to bed." That's me, or it was. Skooby. My dad was the only person in the world who called me by that nickname. Now, I'll never hear that nickname again. As the sun rose that morning, I recall my family and the doctors standing around all of his medication in the kitchen as they were trying to figure out his cause of death. They then pronounced my dad, Mervin Antoine Sonnier, dead of a heart attack at

the age of 41 on the morning of our favorite holiday.
Happy Halloween...

Reflection:

My father died at the early age of 41 and his dad died at an even younger age from the same cause; a heart attack. Life is too short... It saddened me as a young girl to know I wouldn't have my father there to walk me down the aisle when I got married. I am blessed that God provided an amazing stepfather, although I still wonder and I have many "what ifs" about my biological dad. What if my dad would have made a generational change in our families health and stopped cooking all of those Southern meals that we live for in the moment? What if my father would have cooked healthier meals? That change in his life wouldn't have only affected him in his weight, but mine and my sister's weight too.

By my dad changing what he cooked and what we ate as a family, he could have changed the course of his entire life. I truly believe that everything is up to God, but we have some control over what we do here on Earth. We are either aiding our bodies and helping them live longer lives or we are killing them. The human body is simple. We choose to complicate it by adding in all sorts of processed foods, not realizing what we are putting into our bodies.

So what would my life be like today if I had my real dad living a healthier lifestyle? I may never know. Wait, scratch that. I *will never know* what my life would have been like with my real father who died when I was nine years old. However, what I do know is that I will use that as a motivation to better myself. I want to be that woman who turns into that mother who turns into that grandmother who turns into that great-grandmother (you see where I am going there). I want to, and will, see my children, and their children, and their children and so on. I will instill amazing values into them and it all starts by the example that they see and duplicate that can change our family lineage instead of the previous depressing "my grandfather and dad aren't around because they died of a massive heart attack" story.

Questions for You:

Looking at your life as it is now, do you think you're eating habits are good, not good, or can do better? Explain

_____

_____

_____

_____

Why do you eat the foods that you eat?

_____

_____

_____

What age do you think you will live to?

_____

Why?

_____

_____

_____

Do you want to change your family legacy?

_____

If so, why and how?

_____

_____

_____

_____

_____

_____

_____

Chapter 2

I'm Bringing Sexy Back

At the time of my father's death, I had two favorite shirts. One was camouflage and pink and said "Daddy's Girl" and the other was solid black with long sleeves that said "I'm Bringing Sexy Back" like that Justin Timberlake song that was popular at the time. If you have ever listened to that song, I am sure you started singing it when you read this chapter title. You are welcome!

I recall throwing the "Daddy's Girl" shirt away because I no longer wanted to be reminded of losing my best friend. I rocked that long sleeve "Bringing Sexy Back" shirt, along with all of my other black clothes. I didn't want to wear anything else unless it was black. I even bought skater brands like DC and Etnie, which was crazy because I didn't even skateboard. Looking back, I am sure this was my way of expressing my emotions. My hair was even long and black, looking straight out of "The Grudge" movie in my all black clothes and straight black hair. Halloween was over, yet I was still wearing dark clothes like I didn't get the memo to stop walking around like a horror movie.

I can laugh about it now, and I do, because when we talk about my childhood, my husband refers to my younger self as Big Sexy. For our wedding in 2018, he wore a plain white shirt under his wedding button down. This plain white shirt looked like a white T-shirt from the back but when you looked at the front of it, it had my gigantic, chubby-cheeked, "big sexy," ten-year-old face on the front. On our wedding day, I couldn't see he was wearing that embarrassing shirt underneath his wedding button down shirt and coat. I just thought he was my handsome groom in his normal outfit from Men's Wearhouse that I picked out for him and his groomsmen. When it came time for him to take my wedding garter off of my leg, he ripped off his outer white wedding shirt and underneath was Big Sexy, cheesing from ear to ear. Everyone at my wedding, myself included, roared with laughter, clapping and cheering.

I can joke about it now because I have healed from it all. But at the time, I was just a ten-year-old, daddy-less girl who ate entire tubs of ice cream even after a full dinner, wearing baggy, dark clothes by day, oblivious to the problems I was causing myself. Now, I see the issues clear as day.

I was in no way bringing sexy back, but bringing myself down. The foods I was eating neither added to my body image, nor made me feel better, emotionally or physically. I was turning into an emotional eater. Food became the only thing that made me happy, but it only made me happy in that moment. After the three rows of Oreo cookies were gone, I would find myself back where I started. Feeling that dark hole inside, that gaping void, sent me searching for another bag of Cheetos for an immediate quick-fix to the depression that had begun to take over.

Depression is no joke. Whether it is post traumatic stress disorder, postpartum depression or depression set on because of other reasons, it is still a disorder that needs to be treated by a therapist. My mom treated my depression through counselors and anti-depressant pills prescribed to me by a psychiatrist. As much as I appreciate the help from the counselors and doctors, I really wish I would have paid attention to my eating habits at the time. One of the smallest, most basic choices we make on a daily basis ends up affecting us in a significant way. Now that I know better, I follow this principle every day because if I continue to eat bad day after day, I find myself in a terrible mood and my self-confidence lowers. I didn't see back then, but the foods I was eating were in no way helping me get out of my dark days.

Even though I was depressed, I regret not eating healthier choices. If I had chosen to eat a turkey wrap instead of a cheeseburger, I would have had more energy. With more energy, I could have surrounded myself with other children my age and been more social, or burned more calories which would have led to a better body image. Instead, I chose to eat unhealthy and sleep more, which only led to isolation and self-esteem issues.

Another key factor that plays a huge part in how you feel is your gut health. Learning more about my gut health and how it affected me mentally was critical. It answered the question of why I would be in a bad mood after I ate bad for periods of a time. Now, I try to stay consistent with putting good things in my body like lots of water, different vitamins that have varying benefits, and herbs in my smoothies. Whenever I progress consistently, I notice longer streaks of me feeling better physically and mentally. What I like to remember is the word "Emotion" means "In Motion" so we always have to be in motion to keep our emotions in check.

Back when I first started dealing with depression and eating my feelings, it was a cycle I didn't see I was on and I didn't know how to get off. My mom had just lost her husband and she was trying to manage raising two kids all on her own. I do not blame her one bit for not properly educating me on the right foods to eat. Parenting is hard enough. All you are trying to do as a parent is make sure that your kids grow up to become successful, smart, and caring young adults. Many parents don't even think to teach their kids proper nutrition. Some parents have no idea what proper nutrition even is themselves.

The media in today's culture doesn't help this problem. If anything, advertisements make it worse by showing us how fast and easy it is to eat this microwavable meal or how we can always bring this snack with us on the go that is great for kids! Great for kids? Yeah right!

Parents, myself included, rarely stop to ask "how healthy it is" because they are sold on the idea of efficiency. We need to change this approach and get back to the basics. You read in the introduction "you are what you eat." By that logic, if we feed our kids sugary pop tarts because it is easy to grab and go, day in and day out, that is exactly who they will become. Sugar infused children who can't sit still in class and who don't want to play outside. On the flip side, if we feed our kids healthy snacks for breakfast, such as apples and peanut butter or avocado toast, they will become healthier versions of themselves, leading to possibly longer attention spans, better behavior, and more focus.

Healthy snacks and breakfast items can still be efficient and handy for those on the go. It only takes a little time and effort to research "healthy childrens snacks" on your phone through Pinterest or Safari, which will guarantee you blog loads of results. Someone out there has already done the hard part. They have created and tested out these nutritious snacks for kids and tried it out on them. All we have to do as busy parents is replicate. The easy-peasy recipe is already there waiting for us on the world wide web, so instead of picking up a high-calorie sugar loaded snack, let's offer our children healthier choices. I am preaching to myself too, as I am in no way perfect. I have days where it is easier to feed my son some Cheetos rather than cucumber or carrot sticks, but let's make a promise to try to have more healthier days than fatty ones. That is what counts. Here is a starting point. How about a bag of apples cut from home with a handful of granola to go with it? Or maybe even a bagel or biscuit from home topped with peanut butter and banana.

It takes a little bit of thought, some research, and then action steps to change your household into a healthier one. It all starts with you! Yes, you parents reading this book or you single adults with no kids who are just excited to have a family one day. I am excited for you and I want the best for your household and mine. I teach these smaller principles daily at my house and have already seen the fruits of it beginning within my husband of over four years now. When he is away from me, he says he can hear my voice in his head asking, "Will you regret eating this later?"

He was in Mississippi visiting his dad and brothers recently and he called to tell me those exact words. The end result was that he did not order the fried onion rings as he normally does when he and his dad go to this specific restaurant. I was so proud of that tiny decision and it is those decisions that we make each day that compound into how we feel and what we look like later. The choices we make as parents set an example for our son. He has no problem eating broccoli at home when he sees mom and dad eating it. But on the flip side, he wants all the Hershey's chocolate candy pieces he sees Maw-Maw eating when he goes to her house. It is all about the example we set, and finding balance.

Now that I am older and wiser when it comes to my food choices, I know that the foods I eat not only have a physical effect on my body, but an emotional one as well. That is what was happening to my ten-year-old self. I was stuck on this emotional rollercoaster of overeating and I couldn't get off. But this is something I didn't see back then, growing up in Patterson, Louisiana, where we would stop at a gas station and pick up breakfast. If you know anything about gas station food, you know nothing healthy comes from the majority of them. I'm talking about powdered covered donuts and a Minute Maid Orange Juice type of breakfast. That is what I would routinely get.

Looking back now, it is a no brainer when I flash back to those mornings I would wake up and eat three donuts then go back to sleep unhappy. Not three tiny powdered donuts, either. No, I am talking about those large, glazed donuts you get from the bakery either in a half dozen or a whole dozen. I would eat those donuts and down it with a glass of milk and then go back to sleep. Going outside to play seemed like too much energy, so going back to bed for cartoons and sleeping in on a Saturday is what I chose to do. I would later wake up to the sound of *Spongebob Squarepants* still playing on my television and I'd rise with a terrible headache and absolutely no energy. The time would then be past noon, so another gloomy Saturday of eating junk food and cartoons it was.

As an adult, now when I wake up, I try to eat something healthy and vibrant. I know if I eat something that gives my body the proper energy and nutrients it needs bright and early in the morning, I will be more inclined to have a productive day. Whereas if I eat something unwholesome or unhealthy, even as an adult I am still going to want to creep back into my bed, just like I did when I was Big Sexy. Or maybe I won't go back to bed after eating unhealthy, but I will have a less efficient day because my mood may be irritable or I will find myself sluggish because I didn't get my body started off right.

The importance of starting your day off right is critical! It sets the tone for your day, the people you are going to interact with, and the example you set for your family. A morning started off eating the right foods will motivate you to eat a healthier lunch and be more active as well. One good morning full of nutritious foods will lead to another and then a week goes by. Those tiny choices you made as the sun rises can result in you screaming at the end of the week, "Dang! I *am* bringing sexy back!"

However, I am human and there are social situations where my family or friends bring donuts, kolaches (if you even know what those are), breakfast pizza, or some other unhealthy breakfast food and I may slip up. Before immediately eating three or more donuts, or even one, I ask myself, "Did you work out this week or will you burn extra calories today?" If so, then great, enjoy *one* boudin kolache (now I really threw you for a twist because you have no idea what boudin is unless you are from Louisiana). Just eating half of the unhealthy item is an option too *if* and only *if* you have self control. I know myself and I am like a bloodsucking vampire when it comes to food. If I have a tiny taste, I will want the entire entree. So, I usually give a flat out, "No, I'll pass today," if I know I can not afford the extra calories. I don't care how good that glazed goodness of a donut smells, I have to be real with myself and say no if I know I didn't or won't burn enough calories for the day. It is all about self control. I stick to the classic rule: less calories in versus more calories out. It is easier to keep things simple.

In the moment when you are inhaling all of the aromas and seeing your colleagues enjoy every bite, those decisions can be tough. I mean come on, who doesn't want to eat the delicious yet unhealthy choice? That is why I say you have to think long term. You have to picture yourself as that "sexier" you and truly want to bring sexy back. If you do that and turn down those fattening food choices you know you shouldn't give in to, you will look back a few weeks later and see all those small decisions paid off. You'll look in the mirror and sing, "I'm bringin' sexy back (yeah) Them other boys (and or girls) don't know how to act (yeah)." Shout out to Justin Timberlake for the inspiration.

Reflection:

There are moments when I wonder why my dad didn't try to bring his sexy back? My father in his twenties was a stallion and looked so handsome! I know all of the ladies he would meet in the club wanted a piece of him with his long brown hair, tan skin and gold chain he always wore around his neck. I have seen pictures of him from his younger days and I see the good-looking, fit, and healthy man he was. He was fresh out of highschool and played football, which I am sure is why he was in such good shape.

Since his 20s, after nearly two decades passed, a lot had changed. He went on to own his own bricklaying company, but as the boss he didn't have to do as much physical work as his employees did. He was the one supervising and telling the contractors what to do and he was not the one necessarily doing the physical labor himself. He got married and started a family, which might have added a little bit of stress too. And he continued to cook what he grew up eating, and the only things he knew how to cook: gumbo, crawfish etouffee, rice and gravy, and other such high calorie meals. With everything going on in my dad's life, each day of unhealthy eating habits and not getting enough physical activity compounded and added up. It didn't take long before he was in his 30s and he was in the morbidly obese category for his body mass index.

Most people can relate to this, as we live in a very busy, fast-paced society that is focused on making more money and living for the now. We have such big goals for our careers that we forget what matters: our family, our health, ourselves. When we get caught up in living our lives for the now and striving for bigger and better, we don't have an alarm to slow us down. As you are reading this, let my father's death be a warning to you because he didn't have any type of warning. The only physical warning sign was his size. He didn't have any smaller heart attacks leading up to the major one that took his life. He didn't even have a stroke and would rarely even get sick. There was nothing externally that my dad showed, other than being obese, that caught our attention.

What we can learn from my dad's life, and death, is that life itself is precious and sometimes short-lived. We should be focused on spending precious time with family and doing things to make us healthier all around. Again, it all starts with those daily habits that roll over to becoming weekly, monthly, and yearly routines for us. These rituals that we become accustomed to are either adding to our lifespan or taking away precious time. Don't take anything lightly, even the small daily choices of what you choose to eat. You, too, can bring sexy back, no matter how far gone you think you are.

Questions for You:

Did you have any moments in your life that were warning signs for your health (stroke, clogged arteries, heart-attack, overweight)? If so, what were those red lights?

_____

_____

_____

_____

Were those warning signs enough for you to dramatically change the course of your health?

_____

_____

If yes, how? What did you do to change your daily, weekly, monthly habits? Do you have any results (healthy check ups, weight loss, happier attitude)?

_____

_____

_____

_____

_____

If those red lights were not enough to slow you down and change what you've been doing, why?

_____

_____

What could be your motivation moving forward to change what you've been doing for years that is not working (family motivation, live longer to see grandkids, be active for kids, grow old with your spouse)? Be specific! List the names of the loved ones you want to live long for.

_____

_____

_____

_____

Fill in this positive affirmation below for you to read to yourself DAILY!

I, _____ am ready for a great day and it all starts with my

(name)

health and attitude! I will choose to eat healthier foods today such as:

_____

_____

_____

_____

(list whatever meals you have prepped, healthy foods you have at home and at work)

I know that the foods I choose to eat will have an impact on how I feel, how I look on the outside, and how I see myself. I want to feel

_____.

(what do you want to change emotionally? Ex: to feel happier at the end of the day, more vibrant when you wake up, more energy when with your family, etc.)

I will look like _____ on the outside.
(Specific weight loss goal, physical feature, or personal example. Ex: to look like Gina Rodriguez, to loose my love handles, or decrease my back fat, to loose 5 lbs in the next 2 weeks)

I will see myself as

_____

_____

(This can be how you see yourself emotionally and physically. How do you want to see yourself that you don't see yourself as now. Make sure it is super positive and uplifting and repeat it in your head as your day goes on. Examples: a strong and healthy-eating warrior wife ready to conquer my career, a loving and fit mother who sets a great example for her kids while exercising and taking care of herself daily, a busy yet healthy student with strong muscles and sharp brain.)

There are more blank copies of this affirmation guideline located in the back of the book for you to fill out weekly and post them around your home.

Repeat this mantra that you created for yourself for an entire week, two weeks, or however long it takes you to fully accomplish those goals you set for yourself. When you start to truly look at yourself in a healthier light emotionally and physically, then you've hit your goal!

But you'd be crazy if you thought it was over there. Nope, now you take the same affirmation layout and fill in the blanks with new answers. Repeat this process every time you've hit the "new you" that you set on your weekly affirmation sheet. Keep this layout handy the first few times, but then you'll get the hang of it as it becomes routine to list out every goal and every step you'll take to achieve your dream You must continually do so because if you are not progressing and moving forward you will slowly start to go backwards so keep moving forward with bigger goals. Good luck, tiger!

Share your success and join a community of readers who are experiencing the same breakthroughs as you. You can become part of the family at the "I Killed My Own Killer" Facebook group page. See you there.

Chapter 3

Go BIG or Go Home

I don't like to say I am on a diet because those things can be temporary. I like to call it a lifestyle where some days I eat healthier than others. Everyday in this lifestyle, I can either choose foods that fuel my body and give it life, or I can choose foods that make me happy in the moment, but make me feel sluggish later. The second option, choosing foods that make us temporarily happy, is what most of us do. Why? Because we follow the standard American diet where our choices are built off convenience and taste rather than health. This is also why most diets and meal plans fail. We are surrounded by fast food joints, advertisements for yummy yet unhealthy snacks, and social gatherings that bring everyone together over food.

When I was at Louisiana State University during my freshman year, I tried many diet plans. I would meal prep and cook chicken breast with veggies and try to eat healthy, but because I was surrounded by friends who ate candy and many other influences, those meal plans never lasted too long. Then, as spring break was approaching, I would try again. It wasn't until my junior year that I did something drastic.

My husband likes to say I am an extremist and I totally agree with him. To get anything done, doing it big is an understatement to what *I* do. Take my obsession with the Jonas Brothers for example. Your normal fan would go to a concert once every few years and be satisfied with seeing their favorite band right? Not this extremist you are reading about. In junior high I saw them when I first fell in love with them at Blue Bayou water park, where I passed out from screaming so much. Then I went and saw them on tour a year later. And then about a year later I did the same thing.

Well, in 2019, the Jo Bro's got back together, dropped a new album (since they had been gone *forever)*, came out with a documentary, **and went on tour!** You better believe this die hard fan was ready to go big for her boys and God blessed me with the opportunity to see them not once, not twice, but three times in *one year!* I flew out to California with my fun cousin who won me tickets, then my husband won me more tickets locally in New Orleans, and then my amazing husband booked an entire trip to Las Vegas to see them for his birthday! I went big for team Jonas and even turned my husband into a fan.

That is just one example of my "go big or go home" mentality. When it came to going big for my health, learning what foods aided my body and what foods tore it down, of course I took extreme measures. That's just my nature. I stopped going on these fad diets sporadically and I ended the meal plan journey. I decided to cut out meat entirely from my diet.

I was called crazy, insane, and, of course extreme, for going vegetarian. Many people didn't even believe me at first. I had family members telling me, "Girl you were born and raised off of rice and gravy! You can't be vegetarian. Get that stupid idea out of your head." To hear such things was disappointing and discouraging, but I used it all as fuel and motivation.

This was a journey I decided to go on for personal reasons, so I couldn't let what other people thought or felt about my decisions affect me. I started to look at cultures all around the world and the different foods that they ate. I got outside of my Southern Louisiana bubble and started to think globally instead of just locally. I reflected on my childhood of being an obese kid and I realized this is a Western problem for us here in America. We have a high number of obese adults and children, and this is nothing to be proud of or "go big" about. I won't throw out statistics or numbers for this problem in the United States as they are constantly continuing to grow, but I will emphasize that it needs to be reversed. I know this first hand, because I was one of those obese kids and weight is still something I struggle with as a twenty-seven -year-old woman because of the way I was raised.

Why have obesity rates increased tremendously here, though, and not all around the world? While other regions eat a significant amount of fruits, vegetables, grains and nuts, we focused on meat and processed foods here in America. Bring to mind those sugary snacks I mentioned earlier that we love to take on the go with a cold soda. Harvard Health did a study that proved one of the biggest reasons American's waistlines continue to grow is because of these added sugars we have in our diet that come from soda drinks, energy drinks, and other snacks we Americans consume. The American Diet is known for fast-food and that has caused an 11% increase in obesity as a 2019 World Health Organization study reported. This same study reported that the biggest reason America ranks number one for the fattest country in the world is because of a rise in meat consumption. This overconsumption on meat has led Americans to an overall portion control issue.

Other countries around the world are not healthier because the citizens don't eat meat or they don't have fast food restaurants. Healthier countries know how to incorporate fresh fruits and vegetables into their diets, they are more active in their lifestyle and they have less processed foods readily available. In 2019 CNTraveler, CBS News and Business Insider reported the top 10 countries as the following:

1. Spain
2. Italy
3. Iceland
4. Japan
5. Switzerland
6. Sweden
7. Australia
8. Singapore
9. Norway
10. Israel

These countries are the healthiest around the world because their diets are rich in vegetables and unsaturated fats, along with their active lifestyles. Many of these regions still eat meat, but the majority of free-range meat is grown locally. Though most people think of Italy as the region with lots of pasta and pizza, Italians stick to vegetable and olive-oil rich diets which aids their cholesterol tremendously. Spain also uses olive oils and they have a huge focus on fresh vegetables in their diets while they are the leading European country to eat less fast-food. Some of these healthier countries have governments that fund a healthier health-care system and they promote and encourage good health and active lifestyles to their residents. An amazing example is Singapore. In 2019, the government of Singapore handed out Fitbit watches to all its citizens as a way to keep them active and moving. These are just a few examples of the top ten countries that live the healthiest lifestyles and how we can incorporate some of those dietary and lifestyle adjustments to our way.

Many of those people that live in forein regions outside of the U.S. have physically demanding jobs as well as different means of transportation. As our American society is rapidly changing and technology helps us in the workforce so much now, when it comes to physical activity, we barely get any movement in a day. We have robots and machines that do all the hard lifting for us. Take a set of stairs for example. If you google how many calories you burn using a flight of stairs you will see the answer is 5 calories a minute. The sad reality is 99.9% of us do not want to take the stairs. We are spoiled by the elevator or escalator to simply take us up without us having to lift a leg. This is one small change we can make *daily* to take a flight of stairs. It is really that simple. Calories in versus calories out, sound familiar? So take four flights of stairs during the day and burn an extra 20 calories. Those tiny decisions can snowball to make **big** results. If you're interested in exploring more about how technology could be negatively affecting our lives, check the back of the book for more information.

Another thing I looked into while on my vegetarian journey was foods around the world. I realized my knowledge on different foods outside of what I was used to eating *sucked*! What my diet consisted of was mainly rice and gravy and lots of meat. I am talking about boudin balls, cracklins, and pork chops with cornbread for dinner. While all of this sounds tasty and it is what most people love about the South, I started to resent it. I realized that my meals were made up of 75% meat and rice and maybe 25% vegetables.

I used all the resentment towards these unhealthy foods and disgust towards meat to start my vegetarian journey. I would ask myself, "How did you let yourself get this bad off? How have you been eating these unhealthy meals for years and not stopping to make a change?" You know the saying "when you know better, you do better," right? Yeah, well, I started to know a lot more and incorporated all those new health tips into my diet to make a massive transformation. I even researched the long-term effects of societies that didn't have much meat in their diet. The results blew my mind. I noticed they lived longer and to me they even looked younger. That was another huge motivator in eliminating meat out of my diet. If other cultures didn't eat much meat and were thriving, why was I even wasting my time eating so much of it?

So, in 2016 I did it big! I went big in my diet and cut out meat cold turkey (pun intended). As bad as I wanted to go fully vegan instead of vegetarian, I was having some trouble. I couldn't go vegan starting off because I *loved* cheese. For those that don't know, a vegetarian is someone who doesn't eat meat but they can still have eggs and dairy products such as cheese, ice cream, etc. Someone who eats a vegan diet is 100% plant based, minus the oreos (if you've ever been vegan, you get that). A vegan diet consists of mainly fruits, vegetables, nuts, grains and anything else that isn't meat, dairy, or contains eggs. Most vegans don't even eat honey. The premisis of the vegan diet is to avoid animal cruelty, and yes, some people look at a bumblebee as an animal and won't eat their honey. Others look at the long term effects of eating honey and the cons it does to their environment. Every person that has gone vegan or is vegan has their reasons for why with some interesting facts that will astonish most carnivores (aka: meat eaters).

Bringing it back to my vegan journey, snacking on cheese was another habit I grew up doing that was difficult for me to break. When I was Big Sexy, I would go to my local Subway in my hometown and they would call me a mouse because sometimes I would go in there not for a sandwich, but for cheese! The nice Subway workers would package me up some cheese in a cookie bag and off

I would go chomping on some cheese. It was common to find Big Sexy walking down the street snacking on some American cheese, or if I was feeling spicy, Pepper Jack cheese.

When I switched to a vegetarian diet in my early twenties, just eliminating meat, not cheese and dairy yet, I started to lose weight quicker than I ever had before. I recaptured that feeling of looking at myself in the gym mirror and being pleased by the coke bottle shape I was starting to see that I never knew I had. My chubby cheeks were still chubby, but they didn't take up my entire face anymore. It was as if gravity somehow pulled my face down and my head was longer and not as round as before. When I would smile, you could actually see my eyeballs and I didn't look like a fat girl anymore.

I found so much encouragement in my new meat-free body. That confidence gave me the push to think about taking the next step to veganism. I was stunned that just by eliminating meat from my diet, I was dropping pounds quickly and I felt so much better. I wasn't as sluggish and tired as I was before, especially after lunch. Have you ever had the two o'clock blues in the afternoon, after you've eaten lunch where you just feel so drained and find yourself needing another cup of coffee or a nap? Those moments went away for me. Afternoons were full of so much energy for me, which led to more productivity. I wanted to continue to see if my body could keep dropping the weight and could I get any healthier.

When I let go of meat, a bonus for me was I was still able to snack on my favorite candies. Those extra calories that I would eat in Starburst, Skittles, and maybe even a Snickers bar didn't really make me gain any weight because I wasn't taking in all those calories that I would previously eat in meat. I did try my best to eat healthy snacks, but I am not perfect. I like a sweet treat every now and then. The fun part about not eating meat is it didn't really matter that I ate extra snacks throughout the day, and I felt less guilty when I snacked because the calories didn't add up.

Aside from the sugary treats I liked to indulge in every now and then, I learned what more nutritious snacks were. Nuts became my new best friend. I enjoyed snacking on almonds, peanuts, sunflower seeds, and pistachios. I learned how to make Kale chips which are really fun to enjoy and snack on. I learned that they are easy to make and healthy to snack on instead of potato chips. They still have the crispiness of a chip, they have the saltiness of chips too. The only difference is they are way less calories and a lot more higher in nutritional value. The name "kale chips" may sound fancy but they are amazingly simple to make.

1. Wash and dry your Kale

2. Lay them flat on an oiled pan and season them to your liking

A. Salt and Pepper

B. Lemon Pepper

C. Cayenne Pepper or Season All

1. Let them bake for 30 minutes at 350°F in your oven or until crispy. You can even flip them over half way through to make sure both sides are extra crispy.

It is literally as easy as 1-2-3! Since I discovered my love for healthier snacks, and now I try to eat more healthy snacks than unhealthy ones. This can be tough at social gatherings, but I like to be the influencer and not the person being influenced. For Thanksgiving in 2018 I bought a cauliflower turkey roast for dinner. This was simply a head of cauliflower that I roasted in the oven and topped with a gravy. I also brought a vegan jambalaya to dinner. This was easy as jambalaya is a traditional Louisiana dish. The only difference between the original jambalaya and my vegan one was the vegan sausage I used to replace the regular pork ones. Many grocery stores sell the vegan sausage and the great thing is it still has the spicy flavor needed for the rice in the jambalaya. Vegan green bean casseroles and fruit salads are also easy dishes to bring to dinners as a healthier substitute to be the influence in the gathering.

These vegan recipes did not come naturally to me. I had to look up many boards on Pinterest to find the recipes and I had to find the motivation to make the transition from vegetarian to vegan. I got comfortable for a few months when I was vegetarian because there were alot of vegetarian options anywhere I went. I knew I would need some help to make this vegan transition, so I began watching all the vegan documentaries on Netflix.

- What The Health
- Forks Over Knives
- Cowspiracy

I fell in love with books like *The Cheese Trap* by Dr. Neals Barnard and the funny yet insightful book *Skinny Bitch* written by Kim Barnouin.

From watching documentaries and reading vegan material around the clock, this is when the extremist came out in me, my husband likes to say. Many of those literary works do an even better job of displaying the harmful effects on your body with meat and dairy consumption and the documentaries do a great job of making you fall in love with animals too. That is exactly what happened to me. This southern girl went from being okay walking into a local butcher with dead pigs skinned and slaughtered all around, to not being okay with her husband eating fried chicken wings. My emotions, obsession, and transition was so bad that I would cry when I touched the bone of a chicken while trying to be a sweet fiance for my man and just cook the dang meal he wanted.

I became so hardcore and cut throat to my vegan diet that I would tell my own husband,

DePaul, when we were on lunch dates, "You know you are eating a dead chicken's corpse." Or when he was finished, I would look at him in disgust and say, "It looks like a freakin masacre on your plate with all of those chicken bones, you murderer." I was taking in so much information and believing everything I saw and read that I became an extremist. I began to punish my husband and judge what other people ate because of these intense documentaries I was consuming. I had zero balance when it came to having grace on myself and others for what we chose to eat.

I failed to remember why I went vegan in the first place, that it was just to be a healthier version of myself and not to put others down for what they were eating. I had turned into *that* vegan, the one non-vegans complain about or make fun of, without realizing it. A funny side note is that when I first wrote this book, I was on my two year vegan journey and I was an intense Nazii when it came to the vegan diet. I was completely un-relatable when it came to my eating habits and relating to someone who may have been trying to make a transition into a vegetarian, vegan, or even pescetarian diet. Life is a journey and everything happens for a reason at the perfect time, which is why I think it is funny that I never published the original version of this book. Thank you, God!

What was it that humbled me and got me to stop being this extreme vegan for two years? It all started when we went to Las Vegas, Nevada. I was feeling the best I had ever felt. I was 130 pounds and could fit a size four, and I had so much energy throughout the day. My skin was glowing and my hair was long and healthy. Not only was I healthier than I had ever been, but - little did I know - my ovaries were pretty fertile too. For a few weeks leading up to Vegas, I even went raw vegan, which is where I didn't eat anything cooked. I enjoyed snacks such as raw fruits and vegetables, nuts, and for meals, I made sure the food wasn't heated. Even though Jamba Juice and Smoothie King have a lot of sugar in their items, I enjoyed many smoothies and fruit bowls from those two restaurants. When my family ate out, I ordered fresh salads to eat since I knew none of the salad would be cooked. Well, while I was eating raw vegan in Sin City, aka Vegas, something else happened raw, if you can catch my drift. What happened in Vegas did not stay in Vegas and a few weeks later I found out I was pregnant!

(Side note: As I am writing this I find it so funny that if you change one letter in Vegas you get Vegan. V-E-G-A-S -> V-E-G-A-N. When I mixed those two things together, I got the perfect mix of a healthier yet more fertile me.)

At the beginning of my pregnancy, my godfather told me that I was not going to be vegan anymore now that I was expecting. I replied to him that he was crazy and I couldn't eat meat ever again, no matter what. Let me remind you, I am the "go big or go home" type of girl so nothing (prior to pregnancy) could ever shake me. I knew what I wanted and was determined to get that and stick to *my* plan. In my mind, I knew and heard stories about the cravings pregnant women get, so I was expecting them and I thought I would be able to resist them. Never say never, because as my first trimester ended and we were traveling so much, I had no other choice but to eat meat.

This didn't sound or smell like a bad idea either since I was going into my second trimester and always craving whatever I smelled. When my husband would come home with buffalo wings, you're dang right I wanted some after smelling them. Also, the fact that I was growing a human being justified the reasons I should and needed to eat more calories, even in the form of more protein through meat. So, I did. I learned how to give myself grace, realized that everything in life doesn't go as planned, and in doing so, it helped me to look at other people through a more caring perspective lense versus an intense, judgemental one.

Needless to say, my pregnancy humbled me tremendously and I changed from that cut-throat vegan back to myself. Not Big Sexy, but myself. The one who learned balance throughout her vegan journey. I am so thankful I went full on vegan because it taught me so much about my body and I still have a lot of those traits today. I understand now it is way more beneficial to eat a diet that consists of more natural fruits and vegetables than a plate of rice and gravy with a pork chop. I look at the nutritional value of my meals very differently now. I truly believe that we are not supposed to eat as much meat as we do in today's society and I learned this by going big and cutting out meat completely from my life for two years.

Another great experience that came by not eating meat is that it forced me to get creative when it came to dinner time. I couldn't just eat what my neighbor wanted to give me because it had meat so I had to dig into the cookbooks and learn what I could cook that didn't include meat. In getting rid of meat, I fell more and more in love with fruits and vegetables. I learned about vegetables that I had never heard of and I got more creative with how I ate them. I bought books on juicing and pinned every tasty looking smoothie I saw on Pinterest. I couldn't just eat what was readily available and I had to look at the list of ingredients differently. I really had to scan and observe what was really in the foods I was going to eat and if I couldn't eat it, I was forced to create my own meal from scratch with ingredients I knew I could use.

When I switched to more juices and smoothies I realized my body didn't need as much food as I thought it needed to have to be full. I learned alot about portion control and getting full off of the good stuff (fruits, nuts, vegetables) and not cups and cups of rice that would bloat me. I also made sure to drink lots of water during the day and that in itself helped out tremendously too!

That is another huge takeaway that I got from going vegan is really focusing on my water intake, especially when I think I feel hungry. Something I learned is that sometimes we are not truly hungry, but we feel that way. That is a sign that we may just be thirsty, so in those moments it is smart to drink a glass of water and see if that fixes the issue, rather than consuming calories that may not be necessary at the time. I learned how to truly listen to my body on my vegan journey and that, I am thankful for.

Looking back, taking those extreme "go big" measures is how I brought sexy back. The day I cut out meat from my diet opened up a whole new world to me. I started to see my body change, my attitude change, and my vitality return. I had more life and great energy throughout the day. A few of the negatives that came along with me taking drastic measures was how I had a bad view on people who still ate meat and there were not many people I could relate to any more. Some of my friends and family members no longer invited me to special gatherings because they knew I didn't eat the foods that they were serving. When my relatives realized how serious I was about my dietary changes, some of them didn't want to be around me anymore since we didn't eat the same foods.

Over time I found balance. I learned not to be so judgemental of those who ate differently than me. When I found how to harmonize my vegan choices while still being accepting of other people's lifestyles, I was enjoyable to be around again and my family and friends welcomed me back. I am very grateful that I went to such extreme measures to bring sexy back and create a healthier version of myself. Going big forced me to draw a line in the sand and get out of my comfort zone. It made me venture out to learn new and healthier ways of living.

Although I started the journey for myself, I know that I have also improved the legacy for my family. By letting go of my old family habits that resulted in the same diseases and lifestyles year after year (obesity, heart-attacks, etc), I have now set a new trend for my family. I know that the generations to come after me, my children and grandchildren and so on, have a healthier example to look up to because of the change that I made. Going from an obese Southern girl living in a Southern world, to a vibrant, healthier woman still flourishing in the South, but making smarter choices in regards to health is a decision I will never regret. I had to stop living in a bubble and allowing my lack of knowledge to be an excuse simply because it was all I knew.

Reflection:

Even though my dad didn't live the healthiest life when it came to what to eat, he still knew how to "Go Big Or Go Home." If he was the one throwing a party, you better believe that party was going to be huge. That is one of the many characteristics I have taken away from my dad's life. I go big when it comes time to party, I go big when it comes to waking up early and having a productive day, and I go big when it comes to being a parent and providing my family with the best. Those are all great attributes that I have taken away from my father's life.

I have chosen not to blame my dad for what he chose to eat, choosing instead to use his life as an example and a learning tool for me. That is ultimately why I went vegan, to discover a whole new world of fruits and veggies that many of us live a lifetime without even knowing they existed. What is in those fruits and veggies can change your life.

What is one major way that you can "go big" in your life in regards to your health that will change the trajectory of your life? If you are raising a family, the amazing part is your "**go big** or go home challenge" can change the legacy of your family as well. Think about that because that is huge, and can be a great motivator; to think beyond ourselves to our most cherished loved ones.

- Will you do something as dramatic as I did and go vegetarian and then vegan?

- Will you take it down a bit and maybe try pescetarian?

- Will you challenge yourself to get 30 minutes of exercising in a day? **No excuses!** This can even be 30 minutes of just walking outside. Everyday counts. If you do that for 365 days in a year, that is a **go big** or go home challenge!

- Maybe instead of driving to work if it's just down the road, try walking there. (I have a friend in North Carolina who does this. If you live in New York, maybe you already do, so keep it up! Like my mom likes to say, "Every step counts!")

- If your Go Big Challenge has something to do with your diet and what you eat, please talk to your doctor for approval. Pick a challenge that is best for you! What is your definition of *go big*? Title your challenge as The Go Big Challenge on the I Killed My Own Killer Facebook group and share it with us so we can hold one another accountable.

Questions for You:

My Go Big Challenge is :

_____

_____

_____

_____

_____

Chapter 4

P

I am sure you are wondering where the rest of this chapter's title is. P is the title for this chapter because that one letter stands for so many things when it comes to bettering your health, moving forward, and acronyms to keep in mind when you are working towards your personal goals.

The first one I will start with is **Planning.** Planning will save you the headache and calories of just binge eating whatever is available in front of you at that moment. Planning means you take the time to go grocery shopping and stock your home up with fresh, wholesome, and healthy choices. My first go-to shopping place for groceries is my local farmers market or fresh **produce** stand. We have a local grocery stand called "Fresh Pickins" that I love to go to. I always make sure to go there first before I go to Walmart or Target because everything that is sold there is all natural and grown locally. There are no aisles at "Fresh Pickins" for me to go down and buy something processed like a bag of chips or a box of cookies. The P's to remember here are:

1. **Plan** - Know what you need before you go grocery shopping and stick to only what is on your list.

2. **Produce** - Stock up on as many fruits and vegetables, local or homegrown if possible, as you can, so that when you are at home and you want a snack, your only option is a fresh orange since you didn't buy that bag of Doritos.

3. **Priority** - You must make the first two P's a priority or you will just accept anything. If it is not a priority to have fresh fruits and veggies in your home, you will continue to snack on those unhealthy, processed snacks that are not aiding you in your weight loss journey.

Diving a bit deeper into planning, I am sure you have heard the saying that **proper preparation prevents poor performance** (now that's a lot of P's). This is 100% true. We can take that a little further to say if you fail to plan, you plan to fail. This motto can be used and applied to any goal.

That is why proper preparation is so important. Here are some healthy eating preparation tips.

Proper Preparation Tip #1: Eating At Home

This has been a game changer for us and we look at one another and thank each other for holding one another accountable in doing so. Though it is tempting to go out to eat because we don't feel like cooking or a social outing with friends sounds nice, we challenge ourselves to eat at home. We understand that eating at home will help keep us closer to our health goals.

I try to eat strictly vegan at home and my husband eats clean at home, too. Eating clean for DePaul includes lean meats such as chicken, turkey, and some red meats. I choose to eat vegan at home because I know that is what works best for my body. I have a friend who does the Ketogenic diet and that is what works best for her body. Regardless of our eating preferences and what works best for our individual bodies, we both know that we have to say "no" to certain functions if that means being healthier versions of ourselves. Being in social environments can make being a healthier you even harder.

Naturally when we are around other people, we are more tempted to eat what they are having and then lose count of how much we are actually ingesting. A basket of chips sitting in front of you at a mexican restaurant can be refilled multiple times before you realize, "Holy crap, I am full off these high carb chips before I even got to my meal." I know it has happened multiple times to me. I tell myself, "Okay you can go to the meet up at Tampico's restaurant but make sure you get a salad." By the time the salad has arrived I have taken in a large sugary margarita and 2 baskets of chips and salsa. Oops.

Proper Preparation Tip #2: Say No Here Or Say No There

I have found that in order to truly hit your diet goals when it comes to social settings you have to either:

2. Say no to the event overall to avoid the temptation of eating something you don't want to eat. For me, that means telling my sister, "Sorry. I won't be going to Taco Tuesday tonight." I have to say no or else I will get there and eat an entire basket of chips, beans, and salsa all by myself.

3. Say no while you are at the social and go and have a good time. An example of this would be me actually going to Taco Tuesday with my family and ordering veggies tacos on a corn tortilla or a salad without touching the basket of fried tortilla (aka: chips). This has happened only once before because, remember, I personally have no control. Like I mentioned before, I am like a

blooksucking, thirsty vampire when it comes to food and if I see it, taste a tiny bite, or even smell it, *I'm going in for the kill.*

When it comes to social situations you have to decide what works for you personally. Either you don't go to the event and eat at home, or you go to the event and use whatever willpower you have to say no. I personally hate going and telling myself I am going to eat clean then have so many regrets on the ride home as I realize everything I ate. Because I have failed many times and have learned what works for me, I know if I can't afford any extra calories or to eat out I simply do not go. You have to figure out what works for you.

Proper Preparation Tip #3: Be Prepared

Another thing that helps me is having food already prepared. I need you to read the title of this section like I do in my head (cue Lion King Music "Be Pre-pared"). You know, that awesome scene when Scar is crawling through the scary cave with the hyenas and then he ends with those words "Be Prepared." Exactly! So at the beginning of every week, think: Be Prepared!

The other night, a friend of mine texted me to go eat at Chuy's Tex-Mex Restaurant. I don't know what it is with my friends and family, but they sure do love some good mexican, or mexican-like, food. Because I had salad in my refrigerator, I kid you not, it was a caesar salad my husband and I made, I had to stay home and eat it. I didn't give in to the temptation of tacos and burritos because I was *prepared.* Yes, I sang it even then.

Having food readily available for you at home is critical! This is one of the best ways to set yourself up for success in losing or maintaining your weight. When you get the opportunity to go eat out, or maybe you are thinking of your favorite fast food joint because you are starving, having food on deck, as I like to say, will save you! It will be more of a reason for you to eat what you already have cooked at home.

You have to have food cooked or those grab and go snacks ready to go because when hunger takes over it is super easy to think impulsively and satisfy that hunger that's been building up. Smaller snacks can be as simple as an apple that you just have to wash or a pack of nuts in your bag. If you have your lunch already made and on you, it is not likely that you will go get something else unhealthier to eat.

Proper Preparation Tip #4: Simply Be Grateful For What You Have

I know some people who will have food cooked and prepared for them at home but they still choose to eat out. From an emotional standpoint, think of all of the hungry children elsewhere that wish they had what you had. Be grateful for the meals your significant other cooked for you at home instead of wishing you had a Chick-Fil-A sandwich in your hand. I have to use this emotional trick on my husband sometimes because like the Snickers ad says, "He is not himself when he is hungry." I am serious. My husband turns into The Hulk when he is hungry. So I could have beans, rice, veggies and chicken cooked and ready to go for him but he is still going to cry like a baby for Wingstop. It is in those moments that I have to remind him to be grateful for what he has and appreciate the healthy options he has in the refrigerator. If you struggle to eat the food you have already available, remind yourself to appreciate it and know someone somewhere out there wishes they had what you had. Eat it with joy and stop thinking about what you don't have.

Proper Preparation Tip #5: H20

Now sing this Jackson Five hit, "ABC. Easy as 1-2-3." REMIX: "H_2O. Even if it makes you go". Because yes, lots of H_2O will make you go to the bathroom a lot, but that only means your body is doing it's job. I'm no scientist, but I do know that it is perfectly normal to go to the bathroom a lot when drinking lots of water. I also know that it is the right thing to do for your body. The more hydrated your body is, the better it can regulate and cleanse itself. Health authorities say you should drink eight glasses of water a day and I have friends who strive for a gallon of water a day. It depends on the person's cup size, but normally eight bottles of water a day is equivalent to a gallon.

So please, do yourself a favor and drink up. Do you remember how I said earlier that sometimes we eat because we think we are hungry, when in actuality we are just thirsty? Think long and hard about that tip as the afternoon passes and you want to snack more but you know you probably are getting close to your daily calorie intake. Instead of pushing yourself over your calorie limit, just drink more water. As a matter of fact, to keep you from getting to that problem, start the day by drinking lots and lots of water.

I like to drink at least two glasses of water per cup of coffee I have in the morning. That is just to prevent dehydration and to get my mornings started off right. During the day, I strive for my daily goal of water intake. The most widely known rule of thumb for everyone's water intake is half the amount of weight you weigh in ounces of water. So if I weigh 150 lbs, I need 75 ounces of water, *minimum*, daily!

If you would have tried to get Big Sexy to drink that much water, she would have a hard time. I struggled to get my water intake in when I was younger because I wasn't the biggest fan of the taste (I know that is weird considering water has no taste). I was too busy drinking Fantas and Root Beer Floats. What helped me fall in love with water was realizing that I like my water at room temperature. I hated eating food with cold water and found out I could drink water if it was at room temp. So, that is what I switched to. To make water more exciting to drink during the day, I would add fruit to it. Infusing my water with fruit is something I still do today and it helps me get in some extra vitamins and minerals from the fruit as well.

Lastly, I eliminated the majority of the sodas and Cokes I was so used to drinking. Just because they had soda almost everywhere I went, didn't mean I needed to drink it, even if it was included with my meal. For all my southern peeps, this goes for sweet tea too. Sodas and teas can have a lot of sugar in them even if they are considered a diet drink. Try cutting out sodas and discovering what your ideal water intake is and see how that can change how you look and feel.

Proper Preparation Tip #6: Eat Breakfast

Another tip for properly preparing yourself for success in your diet is to eat on time. Breakfast is a great way to get your day started but if you are not one who likes to eat breakfast early in the morning please at least eat something small mid-morning. If you snack on something small in the morning, when lunch time comes around you won't be so hungry you think you can eat a cow. Eating breakfast or having smaller snacks in between will save you from overeating when meal time comes around the corner.

This is one of the biggest tips I wish I would have known growing up. Some days I would go to school and not eat breakfast. I would have to sit through six hours of class and anticipate lunch. I would get excited looking over the lunch menu because I would daydream about eating the hot plate *and* the sandwich choice because I was becoming that hungry. If only I would have eaten breakfast or brought a tiny snack to school. It would have saved me from overeating during lunch time.

To start your day off right, simply prepare something small to eat in the morning so you have portion control when lunchtime and supper comes around.

Proper Preparation Tip #7: Portion Control

Portion control is one of my most repeated tips because I have to remind my husband of this daily. Have you ever noticed when you go to a party that has smaller plates, you inevitably get a smaller portion of food? Unless of course you go back for seconds or thirds.

My husband and I went to an event recently with lots of wealthy, retired older folks and at this event the plates were so small. DePaul, who loves to eat, looked at these plates and immediately got mad thinking "what the heck." I laughed and grabbed one plate and added a little bit of everything on that one plate. DePaul put two plates in one hand and another tiny plate in the other and filled all three plates up. His portions didn't change because of the plate size since he ended up with three plates full of food. My portion size did. When we left this event I felt great because I got to taste all of the fancy hors d'oeuvres that they had from around the world. DePaul on the other hand was stuffed from having way more than he should have.

Portion control can be hard to do. Here are some tips Big Sexy should have learned and applied back in the day:

- If they have smaller plates, utilize that to your advantage and don't make it a priority to go back for round two and three.

- Drink plenty of water before, during, and after your meal to avoid thinking that you still feel hungry.

- Contrary to what you parents told you, you do not have to finish everything on your plate! Set yourself up for success and don't fix that much. But in the instance that you have fixed yourself too much food, you do not have to eat it all. Of course, we do not want to waste, so offer your scraps to your children or another family member. Heck, give it to your dog, but don't feel inclined to eat every bite that is left, or you will regret eating all of those calories. It is okay to walk away. If you can, save your leftovers for tomorrow.

- When it comes to filling up your plate, fill it up first with the majority of the good stuff. By good stuff, I mean vegetables, fruits, and a few carbs. Not everything has to be meat and when you do add those carbohydrates to your plate (rice, bread, etc) choose carefully. You don't have to eat every fancy roll or eat pasta and rice. Pick one and just eat that one. Because if you are anything like me, carbs stick. I have to work ten times as hard to burn those carbs off, so I have learned it is not worth it for me.

- Portion control can be harder in a buffet setting. Buffets are pretty common in the south and my husband looks forward to them weekly. When we arrive at a buffet I tell him like a dog, "Calm down boy," because he gets so excited with all of the different food variations surrounding us. It can be a chinese, indian, or seafood buffet. My husband loves them all. The best thing to do at a buffet is to start off at the salad bar and initially fill up on the healthier options. Then move to the main entrees and if possible avoid the dessert bar. If you want to indulge in dessert, just don't go crazy and eat every desert they have laid out.

I like to remind my husband of the visual examples at buffets or restaurants we go to. What I mean by that may be hard for you to digest, but it is something that I live by. Remember the introduction, "You Are What You Eat?" Well think of this mantra every time you step into a new establishment that you are about to eat at too, "You

Are What You See." That simply means look around at all of the people eating at the particular place you are at, and please do it from a non-judgemental standpoint. Do they look pretty fit and healthy? Do they look lethargic and heavy-set? Do they look happy and vibrant when they are finishing their meal?

I love walking into a juice bar and seeing all of the runners or when I step into a smoothie joint, I see lots of body builders. I look at them and say to myself, "#goals." On the flip side, when I go to an all you can eat seafood buffet and see people suffering from health conditions stuffing their faces with crab legs with butter, it saddens me. Overindulging and gluttony is something that many people struggle with and it normally happens at a buffet style setting. Not many people can go to a buffet or an all-you-can-eat dinner and control themselves. Set yourself up for success and choose to eat at healthier restaurants and steer clear of dessert bars and buffet tables.

Another P that I would like to mention in this chapter that has helped me is having a **Paradigm shift.** If you google the definition of what a paradigm shift is you will see:

"a fundamental change in approach or underlying assumptions"

My simple definition of what a paradigm shift is simply:

"changing the way, you view something"

When I went vegan, I had a huge paradigm shift on my approach to food. I will lay out a few of those examples and they are what helped me. As mentioned, I can be an extremist, so you don't necessarily have to take it to my level, but the shifts in how I viewed food and still do to this day is what has helped me make healthier eating habits.

1. I read the book "Eating Animals" by Jonathan Safran, and this book opened up my eyes to the huge gap that no one knows about between being a vegan or being a vegetarian. This book, along with many other literary works, display the need for meat consumption to be reduced in our world. Knowing this makes me rethink my eating choices daily. This specific book, "Eating Animals," helps display that it is okay to still eat meat but in moderation if needed.

2. "Skinny Bitch" is another book I read, however; this book is very polar and extreme when it comes to choosing what you eat. The author of this book does not hold back her opinions on certain foods so now when I am debating eating even a piece of cheese, I think of this book.

3. Just as I explained earlier, a paradigm shift I use and help others utilize is when you walk into a restaurant deciding if that is truly what you want to eat based off of the crowd you see eating there. That doesn't mean that if

you eat at this Chineese buffet one day, you'll look like the obese people you see eating there. This shift in your mentality is only bringing about awareness, reminding you that if you choose to eat this buffet over and over again, those decisions you make have the possibility of compounding into significant weight gain.

4. This paradigm shift is a simple one: calories in versus calories out. Let's just say I do go eat out. My husband loves this all-you-can-eat Sushi restaurant, so hypothetically, let's pretend I go there and eat all that they have to offer. Well, you better believe I have to have an intense game of cardio tennis or some other form of exercise to make up for those calories I ate. I have to find some form of physical activity to burn off those extra calories and make sure my body is at some kind of calorie deficit to lose weight. If I don't burn all of those extra calories, I have to try to burn at least some so those calories don't add up and compound into pounds added on. I also have to be conscious not to eat out again the next day. Eating out two days in a row would be asking to gain weight.

5. My favorite paradigm shift was the hardest change I had to make. I had to fall in love with fruits and vegetables. Anyone who knows me as the woman I am today would think that this came naturally for me, but it

didn't. I will admit that there were times where I stared at my mom's cracklins (aka: fried pork skin) because it smelled so seasoned and yummy, I grew up eating it and it was tasty to me. If I had to choose a crackling or an apple of course I wanted the crackling. I had to reprogram my brain to learn to love the good stuff and hate the bad stuff. Now, I love even the most basic meal, like a good salad. There is so much you can do with a salad and so many ways to create one. Fall in love with all of your fruits and veggies. That will make it easier to eat them.

Okay, now this is the last P, I *promise*. The last word that starts with P to keep in mind is **Perspective**. In order to fall in love with salads like I mentioned, my perspective on foods had to change. I had to look at junk for what it truly was: **junk!** And I had to educate myself on what nutrient dense foods are. My perspective on how I filled my time had to change too. I had a bad habit of binge eating terrible, processed foods while I watched my favorite cartoon. Or sometimes I would just fill the time eating because I was bored. Now don't get me wrong, I still love popcorn and a movie or snacking during the day. I am just aware now of choosing healthier snacks and not eating unhealthy foods all of the time. So I encourage you to change your overall perspective on everything:

1. What types of foods you eat.

2. Why do you eat them? Are you bored? Are you actually hungry?

3. Change your perspective on food to eating it to fuel your body and not just filling the time or tasting good.

To wrap things up with the letter P, remember that **Perfection** is impossible. I used to strive for perfection in everything that I would do. When I had a project in high school, I always volunteered to run things so they could go the way I wanted them to go. In college, I worked my butt off at my job because I wanted to be the perfect advertising account manager and eventually I became office manager. When I went vegan, I went all in. I compared myself to the "perfect" vegans I would see on Instagram, like Fully Raw Kristina or Johnny The Juicer. I felt like an absolute failure when I didn't meet their standard of what it meant to be vegan. Thankfully, after going through my vegan journey with all the ups and the downs, I have found that balance works so much better than striving for perfection.

Being perfect at something is not achievable or sustainable. I have learned that we have to let go of wanting to be perfect at something and just try our best to accomplish whatever personal goal that may be. We have to be ready to fail because it will happen. There will be days when your willpower is stronger than other days, so all we can really do is celebrate the good days and get over the bad ones.

Waking up with a positive attitude is key. Regardless of what happened yesterday we must wake up with a new mindset and always try to do better.

Now, when I find myself in a sluggish mood or I have a nasty attitude, I reflect on what I have been eating. I wouldn't classify myself as 100% vegan or vegetarian now because I live a very busy life in South Louisiana, being a mom, wife, writer, and business owner. Sometimes at dinner, social functions, or cookouts, I eat whatever is available. I make sure to do it in moderation, and in the days to come I know how to "shake back," as I like to say. For instance, we have a neighbor who loves to barbeque. This guy will smoke ribs at four in the morning before he goes to work and then when he gets off of work from eight to midnight he is making jambalaya or grilling steaks. My husband is one of his good friends and if you do not try his food, it is a total slap in the face to him, so when they are cooking, I will eat a little. Then in the days to come, to avoid an emotional spiral or physical setbacks in bringing sexy back, I will juice, eat lots of salads, and mainly eat at home. That is the biggest factor for me and my husband.

Reflection:

My dad loved a good meal and that is one thing that I learned from him. I have numerous memories of my younger self being BigSsexy and my favorite place to go to after school was the Ryan's Buffet. Many of them have closed down now, but they still have similar ones open such as Golden Corral. The amazing thing that I know now that I didn't know then is how incredible the salad bar is (Aha! Paradigm Shift). DePaul recently took me to Golden Corral and they had honey dew melon, peaches, pineapples, lettuce, nuts, and several dressings to choose from. Aside from an incredible salad bar, they had healthier food options. Not only was there fried chicken, but baked chicken was an option too. There was grilled salmon. My perspective and how I see buffets have changed from Big Sexy to who I am now. That makes it easier when I am in those environments, I can stick closely to what I normally would eat.

Questions for You:

What is one way your perspective needs to change when it comes to overeating? Do you go to Olive Garden excited about the never-ending stuffed pasta when you need to look at the endless soup and salad instead? Or do you snack on unhealthy candies all throughout the day when you need to switch to healthier choices such as nuts, seeds, and fruits? List the way you look at food now and how you are going to change the way you view the amount of food you eat.

_____

_____

_____

_____

_____

What was your favorite Proper Preparation Prevents Poor Performance Tip? How can you utilize that one tip more daily in your life?

_____

_____

_____

_____

_____

When it come to tip #2: "Saying No Here or There," what type of person are you? Do you have to say no to attending social gatherings so you don't eat outside of what you are supposed to? Or can you actually attend the function and say no to the food when you are looking at it?

_____

_____

_____

_____

_____

Be honest with yourself. If you don't know which type of person you are, try it out. If you find yourself saying you'll go to the gathering and only eat what you are supposed to eat but leave afterwards regretting what you ate, then you know your best option is to say no next time. Or if you can attend the function while seeing and smelling all of the yummy fatty foods, but you don't touch them then, more power to you! You can actually attend social gatherings and use control by sticking to what you are supposed to eat regardless of your surroundings.

Activity:

Now go back through this chapter and highlight every word that started with the letter P. Which one do you need to focus more on to help you be a healthier and happier version of yourself?

Chapter 5

Environment Is Everything

Growing up as Big Sexy, I didn't realize what type of culture I was being raised in. Watching adults drink on the weekends and cook a large pot of gumbo was normal where I grew up. I watched people look forward to their weekends and anxiously wait for their next meal like it was going to be their last just because it was going to taste amazing. That was the typical Louisiana culture where food brought everyone and every conversation together.

It wasn't until I moved to Atlanta, Georgia when I was 23 years old that my eyes were opened to a new, healthier way of living. In 2017, as DePaul and I rode into the city of Atlanta in our gigantic U-Haul truck, I saw men doing pull ups on the light post and women with fanny packs and tight pants happily jogging down Peachtree Street. I noticed a completely different vibe in Atlanta than I had ever seen in Louisiana. There were families together at the park, exercising and having fun outside, taking in vitamin D from the sun. The only time I remember my younger self going outside to run as a kid is when I heard the ice cream truck outside my mom's house. It was eye opening to see so many people in the city so focused on their health and happy about it. It was just a normal part of their lifestyle.

As we drove closer and closer to our new home, I realized we didn't have any Sonic fast food joints right next door like back in Louisiana. There was no more Popeyes chicken or Burger King on every corner. Where we lived in Buckhead, the closest thing to fast food was a Chic-Fil-A. What I did notice was there were multiple juice bars on every block and places where you go and eat a poké bowl. I immediately thought, "What in the world is a poke bowl?" My husband insisted it was a restaurant you go to, "poke" items on a stick and then cook them. Little did our young minds know, "poké" is a hawaiin term that means diced raw fish. I was not used to seeing so many healthier eating establishments. I started to wonder if there was a correlation between all of the fit and motivated people I saw all around me in Atlanta and the nutritious variations of restaurants they got to choose from. On the other hand, was my environment the reason I grew up eating unhealthy foods because all I knew was gas station food, fast food, and unhealthy dishes to eat at home like tripe rice and gravy?

While listening to an informational talk one day on iTunes, it hit me! There *is* a correlation between your physical location and the foods that are available there. There are many cultural forces that affect a physical environment, but there are also economical influences. This simply means, where there is more money there are more nutritional eating options and on the flip side where there is less money there is less healthier eating choices. Knowing this correlation really hit home for me because I grew up in small-town Patterson, Louisia. My hometown averages about 6,000 people and we don't even have a stop light in our town because we are so tiny. The population wasn't the largest and neither was the average income. Now, it makes sense that cheap, yet unhealthy, snacks were available everywhere, but I had no idea what fresh-pressed juice was growing up.

This is something I still have to keep in mind whenever I go home. I can't go home to visit my family and expect to eat a vibrant acai bowl for breakfast. The citizens of Patterson only know what the standard American diet says is breakfast: eggs, bacon, grits, and biscuits. For example, my stepdad loves to get donuts for breakfast. I love my stepdad and I appreciate his sweet gesture of breakfast. However, I know that I can not indulge in those donuts every morning I spend with him. There are mornings when I am with him and I will eat his donuts and then there are also mornings where I buy us breakfast. My stepdad loves a sweet, juicy pear and grapes, so I enjoy picking the juiciest pear for him and treating him to a healthier breakfast. When you know better, you do better. If you do live in a small town such as the one I grew up in, you can still do better and eat healthier even though your choices are limited. Whenever I go home to visit, I stock up on lots of fresh fruit. Every grocery store has at least your basic fruits and vegetables in their produce section, so you can always keep it simple and eat fruit or veggies. Adding some yogurt to that is an option, and then you have a fancy parfait breakfast in whatever small town you may be in. Get creative and make those possibilities of healthier food choices happen for you!

Being surrounded by so many healthy choices in Atlanta was a huge game changer for me. And yes, I will admit, this did make eating more nutritious foods way easier. For my twenty-fourth birthday I was able to have a huge vegan cake and the restaurant I invited my friends and family to was all vegan. For me, it couldn't get any better than that. This was at the time when I began my vegan journey, so it really aided in helping me find options that I was able to eat while out with my friends.

Once I got pregnant, we decided to move back to Louisiana. My biggest fear was moving back home to Louisiana, being pregnant, putting on lots of weight, and not being able to get the weight off. The great news is, I am one year post-baby and I'm back to my pre-pregnancy weight. It is not because I moved back to Atlanta either. I stayed in Louisiana and realized controlling my environment is as much of a mental thing as it is as a physical challenge.

Though I went through pregnancy in the swamplands of Louisiana, that didn't mean I had to eat like everyone else around me. I did not have to conform to the normal rituals and routines of a cajun and go back to my Big Sexy days. If being my ideal and healthy self while pregnant was important to me, I knew I had to make the changes I wanted to see around me. Dang, there is no juice bar...I guess that means I have to make juice myself. Oh man, no restaurants around here know how to make a tofu bowl...I better look up an easy and yummy recipe on Pinterest and make it happen. I started to control those things that I could control based off of what I knew and learned from Atlanta. Even though it would have been way easier to keep telling myself those excuses, I forced myself to find the solution for each obstacle.

That is a habit that I still utilize today. For instance, if I am in a restaurant and the waiter says they do not have any vegan items I will overcome that obstacle and figure it out. An easy fix is simply finding a salad that they have and eliminating any meat and cheese with a nice olive oil or balsamic vinaigrette dressing. Or if I am super hungry and I want a more filling meal, I will ask the waiter or chef to lay out all of the fruits and veggies they have in the kitchen and create some type of stir-fry.When there is a will, there is a way! You just have to persevere and make it happen because no one else will do it for you.

If you find yourself in a similar situation, where you know the environment is everything and it plays a huge role in your weight loss journey, start creating that environment for yourself. Now, I am sure you can't just up and move to a new city and learn their healthier ways of living, but I am sure you can follow some cool pages on Instagram that have those same characteristics within them. Stop searching hashtags that say #yummy or #Bon Appétit and look up keywords such as #eatfit, #eatclean or #eatgoodfeelgood. Don't get me wrong, you may find some healthy recipes while searching words with "yum" in them, but I am positive you will find way more healthier things to cook by searching health specific hashtags. We have to be intentional with everything we do, or we are not going to get closer to our desired goals.

Another thing that I got really intentional about is watching who I was hanging out with. It is proven that you are the average of the five main people you hang out with. So I got very intentional about watching the physical environment I put myself in. Think about it: If you have one specific goal and your friend has another totally different goal, can you reach your goal quicker by associating with them? No. It will make it harder because it can be hard to find common ground without one of you compromising to the other one's standard. I had, and still have, friends who don't really care in finding their ideal self when it comes to their health at this point in their life. That is okay for them. But that is not okay for me. I still love those friends and talk to them every now and then, but I cannot hang out with them for long periods of time or their ways will become my ways, their habits will eventually become my habits and their cravings become my cravings. When I hang out with someone who eats out a lot, I tend to start eating out.

Another example is if I am used to waking up early to workout and I have a friend who is not that motivated, not only do I have to force myself to get out of bed but now I have to try to motivate her to do the same. It is so much easier to just agree with her that sleeping in sounds so much more fun than hitting the gym. Then that is exactly what I do and that habit creeps into the days to follow. In retrospect, if I had a friend who was excited to go to the gym late at night, even after we had a long day, then I would get pumped up too. As much as we can try to disagree and combat the saying that "you are the average of the five main people you hang out with," it is entirely true. This is why we have to make it a habit to hang out with people who are where we want to be or better, or at least striving for the same goals. That goes for all areas of life: physical health, mental, emotional, spiritual, relational, etc. If you find yourself in a depressed state, please do yourself a favor and don't hang out with more Debbie Downers or Negative Nellies. No. Surround yourself with Positive Pollies, as annoying as it may be at first, their enthusiasm will rub off on you.

Be sure to mix it up, too. Hang out with people of all walks of life, different backgrounds and lifestyles. My favorite workout type is group fitness. I love taking group fitness classes because I am motivated by the instructor, the music keeps me going, and when I want to quit I see Katie who is like 60 years old still kicking butt after forty-five minutes of kickboxing, so I can't quit until she does, at least. Just because I love group fitness workouts doesn't mean that I don't listen to bodybuilders or those into weight training. I like to hang out with those guys and talk about their fitness journey too. By mixing up the crowd you hang out with you can learn so much about different things and you must apply what my husband and I call "The Grocery Shopping Method." This simply means you take what you want and leave what you don't want on the shelves.

An example of this is, let's say that I am hanging out with a group of my girlfriends who are runners. Just because I am not a runner doesn't mean that I tune out what they are saying. I can still listen and engage in their conversation and take away tips that may still apply to me even though I love taking group fitness classes and I am not much of a runner. When they say how important it is to hydrate before and after every run, I know that same principle applies to staying hydrated before and after my workout classes. But when they share what the best type of running shoe is for long distance runners, I can leave that piece of information on the shelf because I don't need it. Make sense? Great! Now use it in your life.

Rachel Hollis, one of my favorite motivational speakers, authors, and an overall badass mom and wife, is my favorite example of hanging out with a mixed crowd. She doesn't let her personal beliefs and values stand in the way of hanging out with someone who differs from her. In doing so, she impacts that person's life and gets to take away some pretty cool tips from theirs too. That is the importance of mixing it up. You open up other people's perspective to things they may not have ever thought of and they open your eyes to concepts you couldn't even fathom before meeting them. This is something I continue to do as an adult to grow as a mom, a wife, and as someone who wants to be the healthiest version of herself.

My husband knows this about me so when we were in church a few weeks ago, he introduced me to this beautiful blonde mom of three kids. He could tell by conversing with her that she was very holistic in the way she treated her family, so he knew I would kick it off with her from the jump. She and I ended up doing lunch and I discovered that she is very into detoxing your body. I have done detoxes before and I will read Pinterest articles on them every now and then, but I am not as into it as she was. She was older than I was and there were several other differences. Normally, after uncovering more differences than similarities, people tend to distance themselves from a new potential friend, but thanks to the things I'd read and listened to, I resisted that temptation to push her away. I knew that I could still learn so much from everything she is so well-versed on and I was excited about that, so we scheduled a playdate for our little boys. I love learning new things from new friends.

Associating with people who motivate you is a huge key. One of my best friends, my biggest supporter and motivator that I get to wake up to on a daily is my hubby. I am so thankful to have the husband that God has blessed me with, because on those days when I don't feel like getting out of bed to workout because our baby kept waking me up at night, I see my husband make zero excuses and he rises with the sun (sometimes even before). He isn't perfect and sometimes he may get a late start to his day and have a hundred plus phone calls to make later in the day for business, so in that case he will go to the gym at the end of the day after an exhausting ten hours of work. Either way, rise and shine, early or late, he still gets his physical activity in. #NoExcuses.

His game changer has been fasting. On a normal day, he won't eat until after 2:00 PM. That doesn't work for my body type, from what I have found, but I admire his discipline as he watches me and Lincoln, our son, eat a bowl of oatmeal in the morning, then a smoothie, and later he will smell mine and Lincoln's quinoa bowl full of delicious veggies and seasonings while he continues to sip his now-cold black coffee.

If I was my husband, I would want to dive into the food just from the aroma, but he sticks to his fast. He is very adamant about not breaking his fast until the right time, no matter how tempting the food I am eating looks. (Can you say #commitment?) The biggest take away for me is watching my husband stick to the meal plan that works best for his body and not waver much. I am blessed to have a husband who holds me accountable to working out and who leads a great example when it comes to his diet and determination. Using him as an example helps me to stick to my vegan diet, even when I am super hungry and I am surrounded by chicken nuggets.

Aside from my husband, I like to surround myself with those who are way better than me in regards to their health. In 2014, I had to hang out with this supermodel because of my business. You know how models look, so you can imagine what it is they have to eat to maintain this physique. This woman was beautiful on the outside and she no doubt watched what she ate everywhere she went. She vocalized and expressed on her face how some of the stuff we ate in Louisiana was so gross, which I can totally agree with now from the outside looking in. I mean come on! Tripe is literally the lining of a cow stomach, boudin is the lining of an intestine stuffed with rice dressed and liver pieces of an animal, and cracking is fried pig fat! You are asking to get fat by eating fat. That is common sense, right?

Anyways, hanging out with her helped me realize what we ate in the boot, aka South Louisiana, was indeed pretty gross. If you look up how other Louisiana dishes are made, you'll understand more of what I am talking about. Just by associating with her, it helped me break ties to some of the nasty, albeit tasty, food I actually enjoyed. At the time when I was working with her, she was sticking to a primarily vegan diet as well, so what did I do? I followed in her footsteps; when she was with me and a group of business partners at the buffet and she ordered the salad bar and soup only, that is exactly what I did. Or when we were out late at night at diners and the only healthy option was a smoothie and maybe a tofu scramble, that is what I ordered too, even though those fried buffalo wings DePaul ordered looked and smelled amazing. I guess you could say I was being a total copy cat and I don't care because by mimicking her eating patterns, it instilled healthier habits in myself. By ordering exactly what she ate, it helped me steer clear of the unhealthy options I was so used to ordering previously.

Maybe you don't have that supermodel friend who you could follow their eating habits in person, but once again, we live in the twenty-first century. There are so many ways you can create healthier habits for yourself based on who you follow on social media. I know for fact there are plenty of social media influencers who post their meals all day long. Because you know the saying, "if you didn't post it, did it really happen?" Follow their timeline and follow their lead. If you see them posting healthy meals, I am sure they are posting play-by-plays of how they brought that meal to life. Check out a cool meal they ate and re-create that same meal for yourself.

Another cool thing is that if you see the way that person you are following looks, lives, and thrives, and you find yourself craving that same type of lifestyle, then all you have to do is copy what they are doing. That is just a success principle 101. Find a coach or mentor who is doing what you want to do and follow in their footsteps. Success is simple. See, then recreate.

Aside from watching people in person or online, what else are you watching? Being aware of who you are hanging out with and the information you take in controls your mental environment. Being aware of your mental environment is *everything*. What is mentally occupying your brain? Is it a family drama that you are trapped in? Is it social chaos that you can't seem to get out of? Or maybe it is the depressing melancholy of your everyday life that you are just bored of. Whatever it is, you need to question it. And if it is bad, find a way to get out of it. Is your mental atmosphere giving you life or taking life away from you? Here is a great way to check your mental self before you wreck yourself. Your mental atmosphere is composed of:

- What you are reading
- What you are listening to
- Who you are hanging out around

With that being said, what are you reading? Is it gossip columns found in magazines or online that add no value to your life and only insight into other people's lives that may or may not be true? Is it Facebook news feeds that can be feeding you total garbage the entire time, but you are suckered into reading it anyway? Or is it a great fiction book that is taking you to another world but adding no value to your real life? Is it a personal development book such as this one that is helping you get ahead? Or is it a blog post about the top five ways to get ahead in your finances? Whatever it is that you are reading, you need to question it up and down and decipher if it is even worth your time. Whatever you are reading is either adding value to you or taking it away.

Secondly, what are you listening to? When you get in your car you have the choice to let it be a university on wheels. There are so many *free* educational audio options out there for us, such as podcasts, audiobooks, or my favorite, YouTube University as I like to call it. You can learn so much just by searching for it on YouTube. When you are having a crappy day and start to spiral your way into negative self talk, simply put on a positive podcast about "Self-Talk" or "The Power of a Positive Mind" and I am sure that will turn your day around.

If you make it a habit to listen to only positive talks, it will be even harder to have bad days because you are training yourself to remain positive by what you hear. I know the radio is the first option to all of us who hop in the car, but figure out what works best for you as far as listening to good material and stick to it. I don't care if you have your cousin who just got out of jail in your car, keep the positivity flowing. Sometimes, I ride around listening to my Christian music even with my cousin in the car, who is atheist! I don't change who I am because of who I am around.

And that brings me to the last way to check your mental atmosphere: who are you hanging around with? When my husband and I first started dating, he could always tell when I had just gotten off the phone with my mother. How you may be asking? Because my mother is and always will be a worry-wart. That is something that could also be said about me, but like the saying goes, "she gets it from her momma." Every time I would talk to my mom, I would start to worry about the craziest things because she would talk about them.

Even to this day when I hang out with my mom, I have to mentally be aware that what she says isn't always the truth and how she feels should not dictate how I feel. I am praying constantly when I am with her or when I am about to hang out with her because I know she is unintentionally going to get me worried about something. She isn't the only person who is like this. I have lots of family from a small town and they worried about DePaul's and my lifestyle for a while. "How are you surviving with no job? You need to go back to school! You are going to do what with your child?" Those are just a few things they would say. Moral of the story is, no matter who you are hanging out with, stay true to you!

If you are looking to broaden your circle of friends to find more motivated acquaintances, join a gym. Planet Fitness offers specials that are as low as a dollar start up cost. I mean, come on it doesn't get any cheaper than that! Or if you have a special kind of fitness form that you love, like martial arts or cycling, then find your nearest facility and see if you can start with a free trial to check it out. The key is this: once you are there, you have to make friends! I hated hearing this, and it took me a bit to understand why, but it is so true. If you continue to go to the gym by yourself, then when those tough days come - and they will come - you will have no external motivation pulling you to the gym. It is great knowing that even though you don't feel like going to work out, Smiley Sally will be there to greet you or you'll have Talking Tommy to talk you through the workout.

If you are anything like my sister, who is extremely shy, I know you are thinking this is way outside of your comfort zone. My sister likes to get into the gym without anyone seeing her and get out of the gym without making eye contact with anyone so she doesn't have to speak to people. For someone who doesn't like to go workout alone, or is shy if they do go alone, I suggest a simple smile. Smiling to the person next to you is a great way for them to at least remember your face. You don't have to have a conversation with anyone while there, but at least make your presence known.

This can play a huge role in your self-confidence, too. I used to lack self-confidence and be very introverted at times, too. I didn't like talking to people, so I used to go to the very back corner and run on the treadmill in hopes that no one would see me. When I realized that being timid in the corner was only making me dread going to the gym even more, I started opening up to the idea of working out around everyone else. I realized that the thoughts I was having in my head were, "They can see my fat jiggling on my legs," or "Oh gosh! I feel a breeze in my shirt. They must be able to see my love handles." They were only made-up thoughts. Those fears were not real, so I began to overcome them.

It didn't happen overnight, I had to work on this every time I went on a walk around the neighborhood or to the gym. I realized the voice in my head was a lot louder than what was actually happening. People didn't care about me, what I was doing, or what I looked like as much as I thought they did. Once I overcame that, I felt liberated and I was able to focus more on myself instead of what I thought everyone was thinking of me as I worked out. I still battle these same thoughts from time to time, but with practice, it has become much easier and I actually enjoy working out and focusing on myself.

The biggest factor that helped me get over my shyness was my super outgoing husband and gym partner. Have you ever gone to the gym and seen those two buff guys drinking their protein shakes in the lobby and talking to one another like there was no one else in the room? Or those two moms at the cycle bar right by the exit doors with their water bottles and keys in their hands, but they have to catch up before they leave the spin studio? I noticed those gym relationships and began to wonder why I didn't have that. I noticed my husband had a relationship with almost everyone at our gym, but I felt alone as no one even knew my name. I was simply "Depaul's Wife."

It was evident that DePaul started to make more friends than me at our health club. Here is the real kicker; I *worked* at that health club, and he still knew more people than me! I would walk into the gym looking down and barely greet anyone and then scurry out after my workout. That did not create a positive response for me and I dreaded going back. That is when I decided to switch things up, got out of my comfort zone, and started speaking to people like my husband did. I knew that if I wanted to make going workout a positive experience, I had to make this transformation from introvert to extrovert happen. As much as the introvert screamed inside of me to keep my head down when I was walking or to stay in the locker room at times because the gym was getting too crowded, I knew I had to overcome these things to create a better workout experience for myself. That is the only way I could keep the self-motivation going or else I wouldn't go to the gym as often as I needed to. It was more of a mental struggle for me and it still is one that I battle every time I decide to walk into any public place.

I don't mean I walked up to a stranger and asked for their number right out of the gate, expecting to become best friends with them. You don't have to run next to the cool-looking chick on the treadmill and start having a full conversation like you've known her forever. Take it slow. For me, a simple, "Hi, how are you," turned into a conversation that led to us exchanging numbers and getting excited every time we saw one another at the gym. I loved how my circle of friends at the gym grew and more and more people started to know me and my family. Try it out. Watch as one friend will lead to another. This will keep you excited about going to workout and help expand your circle of good-influence friends, instead of your friends who just look forward to drinking on the weekends.

You have to know who are ten minute people, who are ten hour people, and who are ten day people. A ten minute person is someone who you may need to hang out with, but their habits don't necessarily align with yours. A great way to plan your time with them is based on ten minute visits. That way you don't saturate yourself with time around them and get pulled down to their sloppy attitudes or habits. I used to have working associates who were like that. They were always negative in the office, so I knew if I had to be with them I should try to keep it only for ten minutes.

A ten hour person is someone you can kick it with and they have goals that run parallel to yours. When you hang out with a ten hour person, they do not drain energy from you and the exchange is mutually beneficial. They are adding value to you, just like you are adding value to them. For me, the perfect example of this is DePaul, even though technically he is a 24+ hour person for me since we work and live at home together. Anyways, make sure your ten hour people don't suck the life away from you, but add to it.

A ten day person is someone you wish you could spend days and days with because they add so much value to you. A ten day person is someone you have so many questions for and you just can't seem to get enough time with them. This type of person adds a tremendous amount of value to your life. This can be a coach that you pay for, or a family member you are blessed to have. For me, this is like mine and DePaul's marriage mentors, Montell and Kristin Jordan. They counseled us as we were engaged and we still try to keep in touch with them. Anytime we are around them, on the phone with them, or simply texting them a life question, we get so much value from them because of all of their life experience that they are willing to share with us. We crave the time we get to spend with them. Another example of a ten day person is a business mentor and friend of ours, Nate Moore. He hosts business lectures that we call "business masterminds" every week, and we look forward to attending as many as possible. Any conferences he puts together or any time we can spend with him at a coffee shop is worth so much to us because of the business knowledge he is willing to pour into us.

Regardless of who you are hanging out with, they are either pouring into your cup or taking away from your cup. In order to change your eating habits or workout more, you need to associate with people who will pour into your life in that aspect. I have an aunt who is in her forties and she will explain to me, "Katelyn, I fell off the wagon. I was doing so good at working out everyday when I got off work and cooking at home, but then I stopped." Do you think my response is, "That is okay, Auntie. You still look great." Or is my feedback more along the lines of, "What matters is that you start again. You can do it!"? You got that right! My comeback is definitely the second option.

I teach a group fitness class and some of my participants will come to me with complaints about their hip replacement surgery, their foot injury, or the osteoporosis issues they are dealing with. Even then, I don't encourage them to do nothing or not work out at all. I let them know that of course they should take it easy, but that does not mean quit on their fitness. Any bit of movement is better than no movement, so stay active and do what you can do. I do not like to agree with people's pity-parties or have them utilize their least amount of potential. Just like I speak positive and motivating things to others, that is exactly the type of person I want to include in my circle.

When I would do spin class while I was thirty-six weeks pregnant, I had relatives telling me I needed to take it easy and quit or I was going to have my baby prematurely. While some of them may have had my interest at heart, I still worked out to the extent I knew my body could handle. I understood my body and I knew the limits I could push to, so I made sure to only listen to those who were motivating and encouraging to my goal of staying physically active, even in the final days of my pregnancy. The amazing fruits of sticking to that decision was that I had a quick and natural delivery, with no epidural, just like I wanted. #MissionAccomplished

On the other hand, I have a friend who has been trying to get fit for a while and has not found too much success in that area of her life. Part of me wants to be her friend and butter her up by saying nice things to make her feel good. But would I really be a friend if I didn't tell her the truth? She sent me a picture that showed a snack she had made for herself that included asparagus wrapped in bacon. I immediately responded, "I hope that is turkey bacon." I would be a liar if I encouraged her to eat bacon everyday and then be wondering why she wasn't losing any weight. I call it giving you the "real" or "real talk" and that is exactly how I would want someone talking to me. If not, we will all stay complacent in the current states that we are in or slowly move backwards from our goals.

Something I learned from Nate's weekly mastermind class is that the maintenance myth is a joke! There is no such thing as just maintaining. That goes for all areas of your life. You can't just maintain in your health, in your relationships, in your mental health, emotional health, and even spiritually. You are either growing, progressing, and moving forward, or you are declining backwards.

Shout out to Logan Bowers, an encourager, Son of Christ, husband, father of two amazing boys, and business owner in Lafayette, Louisiana who gave this great example at one of our meetings:

> "What if you worked so hard to find your wife. You pursued her while you were dating, engaged and you made sure to progress daily in your relationship. And then you finally marry her, tell her you love her that one time at the altar and that is it. You decide to just maintain the rest of your relationship from that point on. No more progression or pursuing her like you did when you were dating."

How would that work out for you and your spouse's love life? "Yes hunny. I do. I said I do and I love you on our wedding day and that is all we need so we can maintain where we are at for the rest of our lives." I am sure you can see where that marriage will go. If you are not moving forward in your relationship, it is so easy to start moving backwards. That alone debunks the maintenance myth!

The same goes for your health. If you worked out hard for six months straight and hit whatever fitness goal you had, will you keep that goal if you stop working out and resort back to eating what you used to? Absolutely not! You may be able to slack up a little bit but you still have to stay active to keep the body that you worked so hard for. In any area of your life, in order to "maintain" what you want or worked for you have to continue working for it. The cool part about progression is, *it is fun!* Yes, progression can be fun because when you are on the way to accomplishing something great, it feels great. When you hit those tiny goals it takes to hit that major goal, it is enjoyable! Moving forward and hitting those smaller mile markers is motivating and inspiring in itself. Progression alone keeps you motivated and excited for whatever goal you have.

Business success is the same way. My husband and I used to say we couldn't wait until we were both stay at home parents and worked from home. Well you know what, Momma, we made it! We both work from home and it is great, but the moment we stop pursuing that goal, the closer we get to having to go find a job because we slowly start to lose what we worked so hard for. Moral of the story is keep working hard for your goals, even if you feel like you've made it. Another mentor of ours would say, "Success is rented, not owned." All that means is you have to constantly work for it, day in and day out.

Reflection:

When I look back on my dad's friends and who he associated the most of his time with other than his family, it was his employees, my grandfather, and maybe a few of his other "podnas" (his Louisiana way of saying partners). These guys weren't the type of men to go to the gym after work and you can bet they were not reading any personal development books on their lunch break. Their conversations usually consisted of what they had planned for the weekend such as parties or drinking and many of them were not in committed relationships.

I am sure if my dad hung around other men who were hitting the gym after work that would have encouraged him to do the same thing. If he would have started going to the gym, I am sure that would have been a motivation to change his eating habits. Once he got his health in order, other areas could have fallen into place too. I would have loved to watch that snowball effect happen in my father's life.

Questions for You:

What is one area of your life that you thought you've been maintaining, but now realize you've actually been declining in that area? (Spiritual growth, physical health, eating habits, mentality, etc.)

_____

_____

_____

_____

_____

What will you do to change it from here on out and have it growing instead of declining?

_____

_____

_____

_____

Who is someone in your life that you would consider a 10-minute person? _____

Who is someone in your life that you would consider a 10-hour person?

_____

Who is someone in your life that you would consider a 10 day person?

_____

Here is an environment audit:

What are you reading?

_____

_____

What are you listening to?

_____

_____

Who are you hanging out with?

_____

_____

Did you like your answers listed in the audit? If so, why and how can they get better? If not, why and what are you going to do to change them?

_____

_____

_____

_____

_____

_____

What to Read?

If you are currently reading nothing and looking for a great start, join our Facebook group to get recommendations. Some great success books and positive mental attitude ones are:

- "Think And Grow Rich" by Napoleon Hill
- "You Are A Badass" by Jen Sincero
- "The 7 Habits of Highly Effective People" by Stephen Covey
- "Girl Wash Your Face" and "Girl Stop Apologizing" by Rachel Hollis
- "Rich Dad, Poor Dad" by Robert Kiyosaki
- "Outliers" by Malcom Gladwell
- "The Slight Edge" by Jeff Olson
- "The Compound Effect" by Darren Hardy
- "The One Thing" by Gary Keller and Jay Papasan

These are only a few of the greatest reads to help keep you accountable and motivated for overall success! Lots of the principles taught can be applied to other areas of your life, like getting a promotion at your job or becoming a better spouse. Success principles are very well rounded and multifaceted meaning they can overlap in different areas of our lives.

What to Listen to?

When it comes to audiobooks and podcasts your possibilities are endless! This book is to help you become an overall healthier you! Yes, it is mainly about your diet and what you eat, but there is much more that encompasses a healthier version of yourself. What you need to focus on may differ from me. On a daily basis, I have to work on staying positive and seeing the glass as half full rather than half empty. My husband, DePaul, is the opposite. He is naturally positive. So decide what other area of your life you want to grow on currently and this will change as the seasons change. When I was pregnant, I looked up pregnancy podcasts and listened to "A Pea In The Pod Podcast" which touched on different points in each trimester. I loved it because at the time I could totally relate to it as I was walking through that season of my life. Now, I listen to alot of Gary V, Russel Brunson, and other business owner's podcasts in the digital sphere because that is what I am interested in growing in this season of my life.

When it comes to my diet, I love listening to "The Rich Roll Podcast." He is a plant-powered wellness advocate who interviews many other health and wellness influencers on his podcast. The most recent one I listened to was very eye-opening as it gave pointers on how to live well over 100 years old. The interviewee was Dan Buetner, a

New York Times Best Selling Author who is really big into National Geographic and has studied many different cultures to find the secret to longevity in life. I learned of a term called "blue zones" which simply means the few parts of the world where people live past 100 years old like it is nothing. These people are thriving in these areas because of several factors such as walking and biking, what they eat, and even the tight relationships they keep within their communities. I wouldn't have even thought that community and relationships was a factor into how long we live, but it was all laid out through extensive research done by Dan and his team and recorded on Rich Roll's interesting podcast, episode 504 if you are wondering. You are welcome!

Now go back to that first answer you wrote on this chapter's reflection. What area in your life are you trying to grow currently instead of just maintaining it? There are great podcasts out there on relationships, health, finances, etc. So figure out your focus and listen to podcasts pertaining to that topic. If you have an iPhone like I do, there is an accessible application for that and I am sure other phones have the same kind of access. You can always check out YouTube too and Audible for audiobooks pertaining to your topic of growth.

Ready. Set. GROW!

Chapter 6

H-A-B-I-T How About Bettering It Today

It all starts today, right now, yes, like this second. It is easier to put off our goals and keep saying we will do them tomorrow, but what if tomorrow never happens because we keep saying tomorrow? This is not another Annie play or movie where it is okay to sing "tomorrow, tomorrow." Yes, tomorrow is only a day away, but if we keep saying that, tomorrow will be a lifetime away. In that case, we'll never get to experience that better tomorrow which is why *it all starts **today**!* Next time you are about to say "tomorrow," catch yourself and say, "No! How about bettering it today?"

That goes for all areas of life. When you are faced with the challenge of eating what your co-workers want to eat or eating that meal you brought to work from home, think "How about bettering my life today?" You better eat your healthy meal from home! Or after work, when your colleagues are going to get drinks, but you already packed your work bag to head to the gym after you got off... **What about today?** Are you going to go to the gym, or meet your friends for drinks? You better make today count and go to the gym! The bar will always be there, but your health is waiting to improve, **today!**

You may be saying to yourself, "I am too old to create a new habit," or "I have been doing this for so long, it would be impossible to create a new habit." Those two excuses and many others dealing with age and other objections are all false. They do not hold any accuracy because no matter what your age or how long you have been doing certain things, you can always change. Change is always possible and in your hands. I am not saying it will be easy, but it is possible.

Adam Hogan is a forty-seven-year-old man I met at a business meeting in Lafayette, Louisiana. He was originally from Texas, but some changes in his career had led him to live in Louisiana with his family. He is a perfect example of not being too old to learn a new skill or create a major change in your life. In an interview I had with him, he said, "It is nonsense to believe it is too late to get started at the age of 46."

When Adam was 46 years old, he realized that he was just managing his life and not taking control of it. Many things were happening in his career that he had just been accepting for years, such as not being able to hit an annual salary of at least $35,000, and later, being laid off by companies he was working for. Not only was he experiencing these battles in his career, but he was starting to see how they overlapped into his personal life with his family. Once he realized how many birthdays, anniversaries, and holidays he was missing, he decided to make a change. Adam had watched his previous boss go from getting laid off to being his own boss in real estate, so Adam decided to start hanging out with those connections he had. Adam reached out to his old boss, who led him to other entrepreneurs who had made the same leap, leaving a full-time job to becoming their own full-time boss.

Once Adam saw the success, and more importantly freedom, his old boss achieved, he realized that was exactly the path he wanted to take so he could be there for his family as well. Adam began associating more with people who were on that same path. He created new habits, such as reading personal development books, and overall taking control of every decision he made to grow into the full-time entrepreneur he wanted to be. Adam set a personal goal for himself to get this done by the age of 50 and he is currently creating that path for himself. He is still working his current job and subconsciously speaking to himself everyday that he is a full-time land flipper. Even though he is not there yet, he reminds himself every morning with positive affirmations when he wakes up that he is on the path to becoming a full-time land flipper. Adam understands that he can better himself *today*, no matter what his age is.

Adam exhibits some of the best habits that anyone must develop in order to accomplish a new goal.

1. Speaking it into existence! Even though Adam is currently still working in the oil field, he is not telling himself daily that he is stuck there. He is doing the complete opposite. Adam is telling himself that he is in real estate full time and subconsciously that is planting seeds of growth in his own mind.

2. Adam is associating with people who are where he wants to be. He can't learn new skills about real estate by hanging out with his oil field friends, so he is making it a habit to spend time with those who have achieved the same thing he wants to accomplish.

3. Adam is reading, journaling, and listening to new material. He is trying to grow in a new skill set, which means learning things. He knows that it all starts with his mindset, so he is 100% focused on changing that.

4. He is persevering even on those tough days. Adam had mentioned in the interview I did with him that when he gets off of work, on tough days especially, he does not feel like going home to read or study land. He still makes himself do it and is happy when it is done that he pushed through. He understands that those daily decisions he makes in the moment will significantly affect him later on.

5. He is not letting his excuse of age stop him from growing. It is easier for Adam to believe he is too old, not educated enough, or some other excuse. Instead, he is overcoming each objection and making it happen for himself no matter what.

Now, you may be wondering how Adam's perseverance to change his career relates to your desire to change your diet or exercise more. Those two goals are very similar because of the changes it takes to get there. Let's recap those big changes Adam is making in his career path.

1. Just like Adam is speaking his future career into existence, we have to speak our physical goals into existence. If you want to be a healthier version of yourself, it starts by what you speak. If you speak, "I am fat. I need to lose weight," you will not be motivated to do so. Listen to the first three words of that sentence. "I am fat." There is no hope, no

true belief in yourself in that statement, and therefore harder to combat mentally. The right way to speak that is, "I *can* be healthy and *will* lose weight." Now you are believing in yourself and speaking good things which will lead to good action steps. By simply changing the words you speak, you can begin to carve out a healthier version of yourself *TODAY.*

2. Perseverance is key. Just like Adam did the difficult task when it was the most challenging and he was tired, if you are trying to lose weight or become healthier, you will have to do the same thing *today.* This means waking up and running early in the morning before work, even when your bed is holding you tight and begging you not to leave. When you get off of work from a tough day and you want to order a pizza instead of cooking a healthy meal, resist that temptation. You have to force yourself to do the hard task and then thank yourself after it is all done because you did the right thing for your personal goals. When you begin to take on those daily challenges and do them even when they are hard to do, they eventually become easier and gratifying to do. So persevere through them *TODAY.*

3. Do not let any excuse stop you. As I am writing this, I have a personal goal of letting go of two more inches on my waist and losing

ten more pounds. Currently, we are going through a remarkable piece of history, the Covid-19 pandemic. Not only is my gym shut down, but *every* gym is closed. That can be a huge excuse, but I refuse to let it be. I am twenty-one days into working out consistently, even though our nation is on lockdown. I have overcome this excuse by finding new outdoor workouts to keep myself encouraged, motivated, and enjoying the great outdoors while getting some vitamin D. Do not let any excuses stand in the way of you and your goals. Have a "no excuses" mentality starting *TODAY.*

Change is always a possibility in your health, in your finances, in your relationships, etc. And it all starts but what habits we change today. That saying, "You can't teach an old dog new tricks" might be true, but an old dog can teach *himself* new tricks. It is all determined by whether that old dog wants to learn those new tricks or not. So if you find yourself in a similar situation, where you want to eat better because you have been eating unhealthily for twenty years or more, or maybe you want to grow personally in your career but you have been stagnant at your job for over fifteen years, you can most definitely do it!

We need to choose today to better ourselves. I am super thankful that I realized this in my early twenties and started making healthier choices from that day forward. However, that does not mean that if you are in your late forties, fifties, or sixties you can't change anything. I know several people well over forty that have realized that the life they have been living is not one that they wanted to continue. They reversed a lot of their health issues they've been living with by eating cleaner and being more physically active. That saying, "An old person is stuck in their own ways," can be true, but only if you allow it to be. You are in control, you decide if you are stuck in your ways or not.

You change those habits by expanding your knowledge and you can even expand your circle of influence no matter how old you get. You are never too old to make new friends or pick up a book and learn a new topic. You may feel too old to use social media or listen to a podcast, but that is okay. They have CD's too or ask your grandchild to show you how to work "the YouTube." No matter how old you are, you can always find a way to figure it out and do better, *today*. So when you find yourself putting off learning a healthy new recipe to cook, stop waiting and ask yourself, "How About Bettering It Today?"

No matter what your age, race, sexuality, or even BMI is today, it can change tomorrow based off of what you do today! It all starts with what you want and how bad you want it. How do you see yourself? Who do you want to become?

When I was "Big Sexy," I saw myself as big sexy. Back in those days of the 1990's, I would go to water parks with my family in a two piece bathing suit. I remember pulling into the parking lot of Blue Bayou Water Park and my sister would rub my belly around and around as she'd chant "crystal ball, crystal ball," like my tummy was some magical crystal ball. All she was implying was how large my stomach stuck out and that only made me more self conscious so I would drown myself in a large, loaded nacho at the concession stand. I truly believed every word she said about me, including the fact that I was "big boned" and supposed to look this way all my life. It wasn't until I was older that I realized, "Wait a minute... I am choosing to walk around with the crystal ball of a belly because of the foods I am eating. So *how about bettering it today?*" And sure enough, I was about to do so. And the same goes for you.

It is all about what we believe and what we tell ourselves. The Bible says it and I am a firm believer that there is power in the spoken word! What we say will eventually come to life. That is why I chose to wake up every morning and speak positive things over my life, my husband, my son, my family, my health, my family's health, my goals, etc.

In the mornings, I also choose how I look at myself. I mentioned a man named Logan Bowers earlier. He spoke on this amazing example and analogy at one of our mastermind conferences about looking at yourself as either a red folder or blue folder. Allow me to elaborate on his killer example below:

Let us say for this example's sake that you have a file cabinet with red files and blue files to choose from. The red file is the ideal version that you aim to be. For me, when I was Big Sexy, my red file looked amazing when I glanced in the mirror. My love handles were nonexistent, and not a single flap of back fat could be seen hanging out of, or even through, my shirt. My red-file me had a less chubby face and just a skinnier overall appearance. That red file image was more than fifty pounds lighter than what I was at the time, so that red file only existed in my imagination. In the file cabinet there were way more blue files than red files. Those blue files contained depressing encodings of how other people viewed me. The blue file was who I was at the time, which meant the overweight version of myself every time I looked in the mirror. It was my sister telling me I am always going to be that version of myself. That blue file was me choosing to eat two plates at dinner time just because I could and I was used to doing it. The file cabinet had significantly more blue files than red files. So when everyone was reminding me of who I was, the chunky chick, I had to search deep to find the red file version of myself that I desired to be.

Every morning I got to wake up and choose to base my day off of a red file or a blue file. If I chose a blue file, nothing would change. I would still be obese, eating the same things, and barely getting in much physical activity. If I chose a red file, I would be venturing out to unknown territory. This meant

I would be eating cleaner foods that would be new to me, starting to get my physical health in order, and trying to be a better version of myself. Even if I chose to be a red file and instill better habits, it wouldn't matter what I did that day because people would still see me as what was on the outside, a blue file. People would still see me as the heavy-set, creole chick, no matter if I was going to the gym or not. So in the moment it was easier to just be a blue file.

The tough thing about goals is that they are long-term. If I did better myself that day, it didn't matter then because the habits never showed results until weeks later. Habits take time to adapt to and they take time to showcase your results. I read that it takes 21 days to form a habit. Darren Hardy's book, "The Compound Effect," helped me to transform my goals into more long-term goals and I realized that my longer, deep-rooted habits would be the hardest to change. I started to understand those principles, which is why I made a commitment to see myself every single day as a red file. Even when I was smiling at myself in the mirror and my cheeks covered my eyeballs, I still envisioned the future version of myself. One where I could smile cheek to cheek and still see my green eyes. I had to see myself as this healthier, ideal version of me because no one else would. I knew that keeping my same depressing, over-eating blue file habits wouldn't get me to my ideal red-file overnight, but I still practiced healthier red-file habits.

And the same goes for you. You have to envision yourself as that vibrant red file and start implementing daily habits in your life that will get you to that better version of yourself. What does that look like to you? What is your current blue file status? The one that fills your filing cabinet. Are your blue files telling you that you amount to nothing? Do your blue files shout mediocrity to you? Are you tired of living the same old life every single day and seeing no change? Then base your red files off of the change that you want to see. Maybe your red files look like a more physically active version of yourself. One where you can get off the couch and simply throw a ball around with your grandchildren. Or maybe your red file, your ideal self, stops eating junk and has the willpower to say "no" to certain foods. Hold to your red file ideals, no matter how many failed attempts and blue files you have dragging around in your dusty file cabinet. It is time to do some spring cleaning. Search in that file cabinet for the red file you aspire to be and make it happen!

Wake up every morning and repeat exactly what that red file is for you. The hard part is that you will be surrounded by all of your blue files that you are currently living. That means you won't see any immediate change. It is not until weeks go by that you will start to see more of those red files pop up in your life. Eventually, you'll start to see more red files than blue files, but it certainly does not happen overnight. It takes time, willpower, and speaking it over your life when no one else will.

When I made the decision to go vegetarian, I told my husband and his response was, "Ok." I thought, "What?! Okay?!? That is all I get?" I was expecting an encouraging, "You can do it baby," or, "That is a great idea. I'll give it a try with you." But nope. I was alone in the dark, trying to figure out this veggie life all by myself. And that is exactly how your red file journey will most likely be. You may have a friend or family member who says they want to join you on a weight loss journey or start working out with you, and that's great, however, sometimes they may fall off the wagon sooner than you. It is your responsibility to stick to your red file and keep that version of yourself as the goal. Keep striving for that new version of you, even when others quit on you.

I had a lot of belief in myself even when others did not. Several times I would tell my mom or another family member that I didn't eat meat and their response was, "That is crazy girl! You are from Louisiana, born and raised off of meat. You better stop acting stupid and eat." Wow. In those moments, every word they spoke played over and over in my mind, and I wondered if I was doing the right thing. Was my red file even attainable? According to what they were saying, I need to just give up now, stop being silly and wasting my time. But I was determined. I used what they said against me as motivation to push me even harder to reach my vegan goals. I started to form a mindset that I wanted to prove everyone who doubted me wrong, so they would have to figuratively eat those doubtful words spoken to me. I kept my eyes on the futuristic prize and I knew what I wanted for myself, so I learned to let what other people say go in one ear and out the other.

Belief is key! You have to believe in you and the new red-file self that you are becoming, regardless of what you see in the moment and what others say about or to you. Only you can determine what you can and cannot do, so don't let other people's opinions scare you. If anything, use their negative remarks as motivation. Simply add that to your list of reasons why you want to succeed and become that better version of yourself. Some days you will believe it more than other days and that is okay. Some days you will be more motivated than other days. What matters is that the day never comes that you quit. I am preaching this based on past and current experience!

I still have to choose every day to be that ideal red file I want to see. This was especially hard after I finally hit my ideal weight in the 130's, and then found myself back at 190+ pounds again when I was pregnant! Once again, family members started speaking negative things over me and I had to choose whether to believe them or prove them wrong once again. My grandfather told me that once I had my baby, I would keep the weight and only get bigger from there, just like my grandmother did after she had her children. I don't blame him or hate him for speaking that way because it is very common for women to never lose the baby weight. It's a struggle most mothers go through.

Once again, I made a commitment to say, "Not this momma!" So my red file became reverting back to my pre-pregnancy weight, then bumping it up to getting even fitter than I was. Now, I am proud to say that I fit an expensive pair of Buckle blue jeans even better than I did in high school. All because I kept that red file image of myself in my mind and I never let it go. That doesn't mean it was easy. On those days when I was fresh out of pregnancy, eating donuts, (hey, I'm only human - and they were the only things available) with a newborn, it was so hard to envision this ideal self I wanted to become. I would ask myself, "How am I going to be a fit momma as I'm currently eating a donut?" What mattered was that the next day I woke up and changed the course of my actions. It wasn't perfect every day, but I made sure to have more healthy days than unhealthy, and that compounded into the end result of dropping back to my pre-pregnancy weight in one year, even when breastfeeding and learning #newmom life.

You'll see your file cabinet with all those blue and red files and deciding daily which one to choose is a never-ending cycle. It only ends the day you quit. We all evolve and hit our goals or we move further away from them. What matters is that we keep growing and going. We may find ourselves challenged with hitting a new goal and still have those same Negative Nellies speaking over our lives. Growing through those moments and choosing not to listen to them will help you next time you are faced with that same obstacle.

That is why H-A-B-I-T is the motto for life. Not the motto for today, this week or this year but *for life!* Every day of your life you can ask yourself, "How About Bettering It Today?" When I get older and have grandkids, that is exactly what I am going to ask myself when my relationship falls rocky with them, or with my own kids. I shouldn't wait until tomorrow to fix it. How About Bettering it Today? Because we may not be promised tomorrow. Or when I'm 70 years old, I may find myself not as physically active as I used to be, "How About Bettering It Today?" Obviously at that age I can't go join Crossfit or do anything extreme (I don't think I will be able to at least), but I can still try to be as active as I can with as much light cardio as possible. Regardless, the point is as we grow older, we will ask ourselves this mantra anytime we want to start a new goal. It isn't going to happen tomorrow but today, so how about bettering ourselves and starting it *today!*

Reflection:

My dad displayed some pretty cool - or what I thought was cool at the time - habits in his life. He and my mom would drink a beer every afternoon when they both got off of work. Even though drinking is not the best habit to pick up, they did it in a very mature manner. They were both still great parents when they were having their alone time, drinking a Bud Light, and they never let it get out of hand together. My dad would also dip or use chewing tobacco throughout the day, and little ol' Katelyn thought it was the coolest thing ever. Now, I see it is most definitely not. And obviously one of my dad's favorite hobbies or pastimes was cooking.

Can you guess which habit, if he would have changed it, could have added years to his life? Let's talk it out. If he changed his chewing tobacco flavor from mint Skoal to berry flavored do you think that would have helped him? Nope. What about drinking? What if my dad chose to drink Miller Lite beer in the afternoons instead of Coors lite? Would that have helped him live longer? I think not. So that leaves us with hobby number three: cooking. That is the one habit that he could have broadened his horizons on and switched up to help him live longer.

Knowing what I know now about the power of food, I wish I could reverse time and tell him. "Look dad. I know you love cooking gumbo, crawfish etouffee, and all these yummy Louisiana dishes, but they are not good for us. Let's go on this journey of exploring new foods together."

That is why, if you are a parent, I encourage you to look more into the foods you are eating, why you are eating them and are they the best for your health? If you are used to eating a meatball sandwich just because you are Italian, just because those meatballs and bread may not be terrible, eating it day after day is not helping you and your body weight. Or if you are like me, born and raised in the South, the fact that I barely had any vegetables on my plate was not helping the vitality of my life either. Sometimes I would eat veggies, but they had to be smothered in butter and salt. Now when I prepare my vegetables, of course I want them to taste good, but that is not the leading factor. Keeping my foods in the healthiest state is what is and should be priority. It is that simple.

If my dad was around, I would encourage him to look for recipes online that are healthy and not just what looks good. I am sure he would still want to try to cook what looks good, but I know I would push him as much as possible to try something healthier and have him see the health benefits of doing so. The old saying is that a girl is most likely going to fall in love with a man like her father and that must be what I did because, oh my goodness, that is exactly how my husband is! He will scroll through Instagram for hours just looking at "yummy looking food" and wanting to eat it all. I laugh at this because I am sure if my dad was around he would get a kick out of doing this too. The point is, try to look for recipes and meals that are healthy and not just "good looking." Looks can be deceiving and most definitely are when it comes to the preparation of your foods.

Questions for You:

Are you good at forming new habits?

_____

What is one major habit that you have that you know you need to stop?

_____

_____

_____

_____

_____

Now that you are aware of it, will you stop doing that bad habit?

_____

If so, how will you stop? What is your action plan?

_____

_____

_____

_____

_____

What is one thing that you have been putting off that you can say "How About Trying It Today"? (Tasting a new food item like hummus, cooking a new dish, shopping at a new healthier grocery store, messaging a new friend who may be a good influence to you, trying a new group fitness class, etc.)

_____

_____

_____

_____

_____

What is that ideal red file that you want to be? (Someone who likes salads, someone who works out 3-4 times a week, someone who looks in the mirror and is happy with what they see, pescetatrian, an optimistic person, etc.)

_____

_____

_____

_____

_____

What are the blue files that surround you that you naturally wake up to? That is who you are today and how other people see you. (A pessimistic person, an overweight Starbucks lover, a workaholic, someone who is afraid of the gym, etc.)

_____

_____

_____

_____

_____

Now go back and ferociously scratch out all those blue file statements you wrote about yourself because every morning from here on out you are going to choose to be that red file! Regardless of who you see in the mirror today, **believe** in the new red file you are making! Do not let what others have to say take precedence over your life. You control where you want to go and who you want to become, not anyone else.

And don't forget **H-A-B-I-T**

How About Bettering It Today

Chapter 7

Sucker

As I mentioned in Chapter 3, I, Katelyn Foxworth, or on youtube JoBroFoSho, am a huge fan of the Jonas Brothers. So how could I write a book without giving them their own chapter? But this chapter is not just to give credit to the amazing hit song that ran high on the charts when the Jonas Brothers got the band back together in 2019. This chapter is to bring about awareness to a huge killer that many of us don't even realize is out there. These killers attack us when we are mindlessly scrolling down the grocery aisles just trying to buy ingredients to make a meal for our families. These killers attack us in the drive-thru line at McDonalds when we are trying to grab little Johnny's next meal between school and soccer practice. I am sad to say that this killer even takes control of my own grandfather as he eats his Popeyes chicken sandwich two times a week.

Now, I am sure you are wondering who the heck are these dirty little killers ruining your poor papa's dinner? These sneaky killers that we don't even think about are the major meat and poultry processing companies. A few of the big company names that may ring a bell for you are:

- Tyson Foods Inc.
- Perdue Farms Inc.
- JBS USA
- Smithfield Foods Inc.
- Cooper Farms
- Sanderson Farms Inc.

Those are just a few of the major companies in the market industry that you may recognize as you are walking down the grocery store aisle selecting your next package of chicken breast. The reason these companies are killing us is because factory farming has significantly changed over the years and it is no longer what it used to be. These mega-meat businesses are more concerned with how much meat they can produce, rather than the quality of the meat they are manufacturing for their consumers.

We are way better off getting our meat from a local farmer that we know or at the farmers market. That is healthier and cheaper than buying overpriced meat at the grocery store. Not only is the meat overpriced at retail, the quality of it is nowhere near where it used to be, because factory farming has changed the game for us. Because these major companies are focused more on quantity than quality to increase sales, the animals are living in filthy, overcrowded areas leading to sickness. That was one of the major factors that led me to eliminate meat out of my diet. I hated watching videos of the horrible conditions the pigs lived in and the cows were treated with. It disgusted me to see hundreds of chickens squished into tiny cages and injected with chemicals to grow at an unnatural rate. And it made me cringe to see the environmental factors that this overcrowding of animals was causing on our world.

With these major companies focusing more on how much money they can make, they are falling short in staying true to what meat really is. Before factory farming was even a thing, back when farmers raised their own chickens, it took awhile for them to grow into the right size they needed to be to be sold. With factory farming, farmers are encouraged to inject their livestock with hormones to increase their growth rate. Those hormone injections and additives don't just magically go away. Those extra substances that were not originally in the chicken get processed in the meat and consumed by us. We as consumers are buying what we think is just chicken when in reality, it is chicken plus extra injections that are not natural to the meat. It is all happening because we as consumers are buying our meat from factory farms. What are factories concerned with? Mass production! If you don't believe me or want more information on this, check out those documentaries I listed in Chapter 3.

This chapter is called "Sucker" because that is exactly what we are to these large conglomerates that make most of the meat we eat. We are suckers for buying their products that are not even what they claim to be. I am sure you have heard about how McDonalds meat really isn't meat. Yeah, do your research on that one and see what you will find. But for some reason, no matter how many crazy fake-meat articles we read and insanely gross videos we watch of them actually making the product, we still buy that hamburger because it tastes good at the moment. Don't be a sucker! Next time you eat a fast-food hamburger, watch a video on what fast food does if you leave it out over long periods of time. It does nothing. Food that is actually natural has a tendency to spoil, and that is okay. That is exactly what it is supposed to do. So if your chicken nuggets can be left out for a week and look exactly the same with no smell, no mold, I wonder what was added in them to make them do that. Is it even chicken to begin with? Think about it and don't be a sucker.

There is so much more information out there for anyone who wants to eat meat. Just because I choose not to eat meat, doesn't mean I don't care.

My husband loves to eat meat, so I try to buy as much organic and natural meat as possible. I love buying him grass fed cow and lamb meat at the farmers market, whenever I can find a farmer who still takes care of his animals the good-old fashion way. Trust me, it is way better than my hubby eating meat with all of those added chemicals from a factory farm. I will not let him or myself be a sucker to these big businesses in the meat industry. Because I know what they do, I choose to do better. I know that the meat that they serve is not optimum and what it used to be, so I choose not to eat it. Just like any business, I am sure their main focus is money which is why the quality is decreasing.

All I am saying is don't be a sucker! Don't buy the two for one special just because the sign says so and you think it is a good deal. Do your research and find smarter, healthier ways to buy your meat if you are going to eat meat. While you are researching what meats to buy, research how much meat we actually need as humans. You will be surprised in that arena too, because most of us eat way more meat than we need. One of my favorite books recommends doing "meatless Mondays" and if we would do more of those, we would be saving our environment in many ways, as well as our health. So stop being a sucker for meat and the meat market propaganda and do your research. Then take action next time you are planning your next trip to the grocery store and don't just mindlessly buy things, buy them because they are good for you!

Reflection:

My dad was a Southern Louisiana man who grew up killing his own food or buying it from a local butcher. In my father's time, these large meat industries weren't as big of a deal as they are now. Where my dad lived, if they were eating turtle soup (yes, turtle soup) it was because they killed the turtle themselves. So they saw the game from when it was alive to when it was served at the dinner table. There was no error or room to inject the meat with something he didn't know.

However, as my dad grew up, he moved out of the small town where he lived and into a new neighborhood. One where he didn't have the space or the time to create his own livestock. He most definitely did for his fruits and veggies, as that is one of my favorite memories with my father: his garden. But he couldn't have the animals as well. That led to my dad shopping at a grocery store and he would buy whatever meat was available and sometimes on sale.

One thing I wish my dad would have done was hunt most of his meat instead of purchasing it. Some of my dad's family hunts their own game, gets it slaughtered and packaged and they live off of that all year long. I wonder if my dad had been more conscious with the meats he chose to eat, if he would still be around. This thought comes to my mind a lot because the majority of the meals my dad cooked involved lots of red meat or pork. Pork chops and bacon are two meats that can clog arteries the most! When I think of my dad living past his forties, it is in no way, shape, or form my dad being vegan like me. That is entirely out of the question. But I *can* envision my father eating more chicken and leaner meats. If only he knew better. That is a huge factor in why I choose to live my life better, making healthier eating choices in honor of him.

Questions for You:

Have you been a sucker for these major companies, buying whatever meat they put out there without doing your own research?

_____

_____

_____

_____

_____

How can you choose to buy healthier options? (Ex. Meatless Mondays, Impossible Burger, Farmers Market locally grass fed animals.)

_____

_____

_____

_____

_____

Do you think you eat too much meat? If so, how can you cut back?

_____

_____

_____

_____

_____

What is one dish that you can bring to the next holiday dinner that includes more fresh vegetables and herbs than meat?

_____

_____

_____

_____

_____

What is one meal that you normally eat that you can cut out the meat in it or substitute it for something else? (Ex. I have a friend who uses meatless ground crumbles in her lasagna and spaghetti)

_____

_____

_____

_____

Chapter 8

WHY Him

At the age of 10, it was extremely tough to look at other kids my age having the time of their life with both of their parents. I saw the bonds that children had with their dads and the cool stuff that they got to do together. My friends would go hunting, camping, and biking with their dads. I sort of envied that about them. The straw that broke the camel's back was when one of my classmates (I guess you could say she was my nemesis in elementary school and junior high school) said something that verbally hit me in the gut when I was going through these tough times.

We were arguing about something childish I am sure, I can't remember the dispute details, during class and she ended the argument with, "At least I have a daddy, Katelyn! I have two of them." She meant she had a real father who was alive and her stepdad that took care of her. Man, oh man, do I still feel that boiling sensation I felt when I wanted to rip her head off in that moment. Since I was on the honor roll in school and a good student, all I could do was kick the back of her chair in the classroom in that painful moment she spoke those words to me. Then after I got off the bus that afternoon, I stuffed my face with an entire pack of oreos when I got home to cope with my feelings of hurt, anger, and disgust.

So there I was at a young age, dealing with the loss of my father and not having my peers there to help me through it. I would find myself questioning God, "Why him?" Why did God have to take my father? It wasn't fair in my ten year old mind how I had no daddy anymore, but my classmates and friends still did. I didn't understand it and had a hard time coping with it.

It wasn't until I was older that I came to terms with the loss of my father. Rachel Hollis, an amazing writer, business owner, and motivational speaker said at one of her speaking engagements that there may not be a reason for everything, but we can find a reason for everything. That still hits home for me. I don't like to say my dad died and there is a reason for it. However, I do believe I can find a reason for it.

That is why I like to reflect on his life and instead of being mad for all of the unhealthy diet choices he made, I would rather use that as a learning tool for myself and most importantly others. My dad's life and his father's life are not a waste, but lives that I like to learn from and use to help others learn from.

I use my dad's death as my motivation, or in other words my "why." Having a why is a huge factor in achieving any goal. There are plenty of success and personal development books for business that illustrate the force behind having a "why." Having a why factor is instrumental to achieving your goal because it is what puts emotion behind your goal. Your "why" is what is going to wake you up in the morning when your body screams at you that you are too tired. Your "why" is going to be the willpower you need to eat your salad when you are surrounded by chicken wings and french fries. Your "why" is going to be that extra push you need to learn and cook new recipes when you are too tired to even cook the usual that you are used to whipping up.

The thing about your "why" is that it has to be bigger than you. Your reason has to be extreme in a sense. It can't be your average goal of "I just want to lose weight to look good," or "my husband is my why." Your why has to be specific and evoke a major emotion out of you now and forever. A better version of the two prior examples are:

- I want to lose 50 lbs. to maintain a healthy weight and gain self-confidence when looking at myself.

- My husband has overcome cancer, so if he can push through those trying times, I know I can eat better and live a healthier life with and for him.

My why started developing at a very young age. I have been missing a gigantic part of my life since 2001; my dad. Ever since then, I tried to make him proud in every way, as people would tell me he is smiling down at me from heaven. Regardless whether he is truly watching me or not, my why is to live a long and meaningful life for and in memory of him. I want to learn from his mistakes, whether he knew they were errors in his life or not. That helps me feel as though, in a sense, he is still alive and his life is not wasted. My goal is to have his story - as well as mine - impact the lives of others by bringing awareness to people's health and how the choices we make daily affect the longevity of our lives. In a nutshell, my "why" is to utilize my dad's life to impact my life, my family, and other people's lives. I want to have a positive impact on other people by bringing about awareness to their health with action steps to help them change areas they may need help in.

Anytime I think of my why, I get emotional because it is attached to my deceased father, who I have so many fond memories of. On the other hand, it is emotional because of how big of a goal it is, not only for myself, but for the greater good, for the people I want it to reach who need their eyes opened to how they are living their lives, stuck in unhealthy habits, big or small. My reason is not just about me, but about bettering other people's lives. I know that if I can reach a stressed out father who is overweight, I can help another little girl not lose her daddy as I lost mine. If I can hang on to my "why" and use it to motivate me, I am certain it will save the life of a parent who deserves to spend more time with their family.

Maybe that parent just wasn't aware of the harm they were doing to their body by the small choice in their mind of what to eat. Maybe that parent doesn't see a way out or know how to eat better. Maybe that parent, even knowing the difference between healthy and not, didn't really think about the possibility of not being there for their child. I know that my motivation and writing this book can change that for them. There are many things and several reasons for my "why" and because it is backed up by so much passion and feelings from me, I refuse to let it go!

My "why" is something that has evolved over the years. As a young child, I had the passion to do something great. I just didn't know what I wanted to do specifically. Even after my father had passed, I never put two and two together and I still didn't have a reason for what I wanted to do. That is because the pieces of the puzzle were still being laid out for me. It took a few years for me to grow up and go through some things before I could look back and realize that everything in my life happened for a reason. Once my "why" was formed, it was solid. Over the years it has slightly changed, but the core of it remains the same. The two biggest changes in my reasons for doing what I do is the husband I get to share it with and the children I get to lead in doing so. Those are two new additions to my "why" that make it even stronger..

Once you find your "why," it can get bigger as each year of your life goes by and things change. Those updates in your life can be new additions to your reasons and motives and they will make your why that much stronger. In my early twenties, I didn't think my why could get any stronger, but then I found my husband. He motivates me so much everyday that I can't lose. When we had our son, it gave me an even bigger reason to push through challenging times. I can imagine as we have more kids that my why and motivation in life will only become more powerful. That is the way it should be! I encourage you to dig deep to discover what your why truly is. Not a surface level reason that you just tell yourself to answer that question, or based on self-esteem, or a worry over what other people think. No, those aren't strong enough to really encourage change. Make sure your "why" is deeply rooted, meaningful, and tremendously impactful to your *heart.*

To truly discover your "why," you are going to have to take an overall look at your life, where you are at now and what has gotten you there. You are most importantly going to have to look towards the future too and see what is going to get you moving during those tough moments in your life. Is it your kids? Is it your grandkids? Is it your life's purpose or the emotional ties you have to your career or business? Once you find that answer, try to dig a little bit deeper and see if you can unlock another level to it. Specifically what about your children or grandchildren do you feel so passionately about? Maybe it is having a full lifetime to spend with them because you weren't given that time with your parents. Maybe your job is more than just a position to you and it is a way for you to impact someone's life every single day. Whatever your reasoning is, be sure to be specific and not something that changes by the day. Your "why" should be solid and strike enthusiasm from you every time you think of it, even if that is a hundred times a day. If your "why" is truly "*your* why," there will be power behind it and it will never get old, no matter how many times you think of it.

Nobody else needs to understand it. Your motivation in life is for you and you only. You can certainly share it with someone, but don't get discouraged when they don't share the same amount of joy as you do when you reveal it to them. Even your spouse may not be as worked up about your "why" as you. They have their own motivations in life that don't necessarily line up exactly to yours even though you share the same life together now that you are married. I know this from personal experience. My husband understands my "why" and he believes in it, but my "why" is not what wakes him up excited in the mornings. It is *his* "why" that has the power to pump him up. So be ready to share where your hunger in life comes from and don't expect others to be as equally as excited as you are. Not even your own mom will be as excited as you, and that is okay.

I can't pick *your* why for you, but I can recommend reading more books on how to find your why and reflecting on your life and what you feel is important. This can truly change the trajectory of your life in many different areas, not just health, if you really figure out "your why" and utilize it to help you excel in all areas of life. When you unravel this, you will discover purpose in numerous areas which will motivate you and snowball into overall success in your life.

A great book to help you find your "why" is a book titled (get this) "Find Your Why." Catchy title isn't it? The author of this book, Simon Sinek, is famous for the power of unleashing potential in many people through "why power," so I encourage you to pick this book up next. There are many gurus and coaches out there too that can help you discover your true purpose and "why." My favorite one that comes to mind is Tony Robbins. Even though I have never met Mr. Robbins in person, I have watched his incredible Netflix documentary, "I Am Not Your Guru." That is an impactful movie to watch if you let it be. And if you want to dig even deeper, go to one of the events he puts on. Your socks will forever be blown off and you will not go home the same way you arrived at his function. If you want to take baby steps onto that personal development journey instead of jumping right into an event, Tony Robbins also has great books that will help you do lots of deep self-reflection, along with great motivational videos on YouTube. Regardless of how you choose to look inward to bring out your why, there is no excuse for you not to do it.

My "why" is directly related to my health because of my father losing his life to a heart-attack. If I truly want to impact other people's lives and do something great with my life, how can I afford to eat bad or live an unhealthy life? I can't because other people's lives are at stake and attached to my why. I saw the life my father lived and how every small choice he made of what to eat daily compounded into such a tragic ending. My motivation is to not travel down the road that he went down by unintentionally neglecting his health, just as his own father did, resulting in them dying at such an early age. The reason I have to keep my health in order is because of how I saw him leave this world so soon, and because I want to use his story to impact other people who are living their lives unconsciously eating whatever is convenient for them and slowly killing themselves.

Now I know that there is a tiny percentage out there for another reason of my dad having a heart attack. And there may be an even smaller percentage for his dad dying of a heart attack too. Regardless, when you look at the risk factors for why people have clogged arteries that stop the blood flow to the heart, those risk factors include what is listed below. The factors listed below in bold are the ones that impacted my father directly. The factors that are underlined are the ones that I can control when it comes to them applying to my own life.

- Age
- **Tobacco**
- Diabetes
- **High Blood Pressure**
- **High Cholesterol**
- **Obesity**
- **Metabolic Syndrome**
- **Family History**
- Lack of Physical Activity
- Stress
- Drug Use
- An Auto-immune Condition

- A History of Preeclampsia

Ten out of the twelve risk factors we as individuals can control. We can lose weight if we are obese (most cases) or we can choose to not let it get that far. We can watch out for metabolic syndrome by being on top of our high blood pressure, high sugar, and obesity. Just as one unhealthy habit leads to another, being diagnosed with one risk factor makes it easier to get another. Many of these risk factors intertwine and work together. I can choose to stay away from tobacco and not use drugs. I can look out for my cholesterol levels and high blood pressure by watching the foods that I eat. I can avoid the risk factor of "lack of physical activity" by being physically active. It really is that simple, the problem is just that most of us don't pay attention to these signs and symptoms until it is too late.

Looking at those risk factors and seeing that I can control the majority of them, it encourages me to take the reins and do what I can to prevent this from happening to myself. That is why I truly believe that I have killed my father's killer. Like I mentioned in a previous chapter, when you know better you do better. So why would I wait? Why should I live the traditional Louisiana lifestyle where you eat high-sodium crawfish every weekend or gumbo that is full of cholesterol and drink beer or smoke? Why would I add unhealthy habits to my life if I know I have a family history of heart disease and heart attacks. I have to take the killer head on and do what I know is right for my body. At the end of my life, whether it be when I am fifty or a hundred, at least I can say I tried. And with my attempt, I am sure it will help other people live a healthier lifestyle too.

Killing my dad's killer isn't something I can do one time and then be over with it. It is something that I have to work at day in and day out. Killing my dad's killer takes daily discipline and there are times when I fall short, but because my "why" is so strong, I hop back on the horse and keep moving forward, and your why will help you do the same.

Chapter 9

K-I-S-S

Yay! You made it to the final chapter of "I Killed My Father's Killer." I am sure by now you have guessed that my father's killer was a heart attack, heart disease, clogged arteries leading to no blood flow, bad eating habits, etc. If you guessed any of those or something along those lines, then you are correct! By gaining control of my health, physical activity, depression, and so much more, I truly feel as though I have killed his killer! I get to live a joyous life for him, in memory of him, and in honor of him by learning from his mistakes. The best part is that I get to pay it forward to you by sharing his life's mistakes and how I have learned from it all to live a happier and healthier life.

Since I have paid it forward to you by sharing so many personal stories, struggles and achievements, all I ask is that you KISS. No, I don't need a smooch-a-roo from you as I am sure my husband wouldn't like that. What I ask is for you to remember that when it comes to your overall health, Keep It Simple Silly! Always keep it simple by remembering each trick and tip I laid out for you in the previous chapters.

When you find yourself spiraling mentally and going through a tough time, just remember to keep it simple. A lot of the time, our mental battles feel so much worse than what they really are. We just think they are huge because they're stuck in our heads until we take control of them. Keep it simple when you are going through a mentally tough issue and talk to a friend. By simply saying it outloud, you can begin to realize the problem you had in your head was one that you were making bigger than it actually is. Or maybe you have a problem with someone else who has offended you. That happens to me and my husband all the time. I like to keep it simple and just apologize. Then we are able to move forward and work things out.

Like I mentioned at the beginning of the book, depression can play a huge part in how much you eat, and what you eat can circle back to how you feel. That is why taking control of your feelings is so important, not just for your mental health, but for your body in general. Trust me, when you feel better mentally and have clarity in your relationships and in your life, you will be more likely to work out physically too. Always remember: a good mood leads to a good day.

I like to keep it simple when it comes to my meal choices too. There are days where I don't know what to eat. Those are the days when I am tempted to eat fast food. I have to remind myself to keep it simple and eat something at home. It is more than likely that I have enough ingredients and food choices to make a complete meal. That happened this week and three times out of the week I ate my brown rice I had stored away. I ate some seasoned and sauteed tofu with that rice and some green lentils I needed to cook anyways. Rice, beans, and tofu is a prime example of tasty, healthy, and simple. I substituted the tofu with chicken breast for my husband and we had one healthy and happy household.

I can even break it down even simpler than that! Some mornings I don't feel like eating my usual oatmeal and fruit, so I just fix a smoothie. I have had friends ask how I make a smoothie and I love you friends, but that is a silly question. It is as simple as throwing some fruit into a blender. Just start doing it and you will figure out which ones you love and which ones you don't. As I am typing this chapter I am sipping on my supper, a bomb peanut butter banana smoothie I made for dinner after I fixed my boys some chicken salad sandwiches.

Smoothies are as simple as it can get. A smoothie tip is to make sure you have a base (milk, almond milk, yogurt, ice cream, etc.) then add some fruit (banana, strawberry, blueberry, etc.) and you can add extra proteins or veggies (kale, spinach, etc.). The veggies are optional and will add more nutrients to your sweet smoothie. You can get fancy and make it a protein smoothie by adding some supplement or protein powder, but that is optional. When I make smoothies in the morning for my son and I to share, I leave out the protein powder and I load it with fruits and veggies. I like to add other healthy things to my smoothie that you can't really taste such as flax seeds, chia seeds, turmeric powder, and ginger.

The last way I will encourage you to keep it simple is in your physical movement too. You know that meme of Chan from "The Hangover" and he asked, "But *did* you die" in regards to him being a bad driver? I hope you have seen that meme, if not check it out because it is one of my faves. But we should ask ourselves those questions everyday in comparison to our health. Not did you die but we should ask, "But did you move today?" It truly is that simple. At the end of the day, ask yourself if you moved around for at least thirty minutes today. You don't have to have spent two hours in the gym to have a good workout. Thirty minutes a day of walking compounded over numerous days will add up to great cardiovascular health. We can each strive for that daily move goal of thirty minutes a day whether it is walking outside, walking during our lunch break to meet a friend, a bicycle ride in the morning, or whatever thirty minutes of activity means to you.

So remember to Keep It Simple Silly in your physical health, your eating choices, and your overall health and happiness. It doesn't have to be as hard as we make it on ourselves people. Ultimately I have to KISS to kill my father's killer, and the same goes for you!

Bonus Chapter

Exclusive Details on My Vegan Journey and How It All Began

Going vegan for me was something I had never thought of previously. One day, the thought hit me and I refused to let it go. The thought was, "What if I went vegetarian." I had this thought because I realized after I would eat meat, I felt heavier. I loved the feeling after I would just finish eating a salad or a Chipotle bowl with no meat. I was full, yet I still felt like my light self. At the time I thought this, I was working as a caretaker forty plus hours a week and attending LSU to get my degree in Mass Communications, so this thought was just a wonder in my mind for one day.

The next day I woke up and I said, "No more excuses. Let's do it!" It was a difficult time because the great flood of Baton Rouge had just hit a day or two before. What that meant for me was that my client and really good friend, Hannah, needed my help more than ever. Since I was her caretaker, my duty was to take care of her daily needs: feed her, change her, bring her on outings, take her to doctors appointments, etc.

This particular flood that happened in 2016 wiped out everything in Hannah's home, including her motorized wheelchair and many other things that we utilized in her home to make living life with cerebral palsy easier. Hannah, her mom, and her dad had to move into a hotel for many months so construction workers and family members could get their home back together and make it livable once again after such a catastrophic phenomenon. I knew that I had to go from working more than forty hours with Hannah, still managing school, sustaining this new vegetarian diet I started, and adding more hours on the road to help Hannah and her family out. Was this even possible?

I never back down from a challenge, so I was willing to make a way to create all of this for myself. I was going to keep up my grades in school to maintain my scholarships at LSU. I was going to continue eating vegetarian, no matter how many free meals were offered to me. If they didn't fit the criteria, I would have to turn them down, even as a broke college student. I was willing to make a way to work those extra hours to help Hannah and her family out while still finding time to work out and take care of my own physical health. I remember this being one of the toughest times of my life and breaking down at the church alter one day when I went up for prayer. I usually never go up for prayer when the pastor says to, but for some reason Hannah wanted to go, so I pushed her in her wheelchair there and I ended up crying and praying with a church member. I didn't realize how stressed out I was until I voiced it all to the prayer team member.

However, I pushed through those tough weeks and continued my vegetarian journey. Remember in chapter four how I mentioned perfection is not a real thing. This was the season that I learned that lesson, because there were days where I didn't pack my own lunch and I struggled to find vegetarian options. Some days I didn't have enough money to purchase them for myself while I was working. That meant I did the inevitable. Yes, I did cave in and eat whatever was available. After making those mistakes on my vegetarian journey I didn't say, "Oh man. I ate meat. I guess I am not a true vegetarian so let me quit now." No way, José! I shook those errors off and tried harder the next day. I learned that being perfect, or even trying to be perfect, can be so almost impossible, and we have to learn to give ourselves grace. Giving grace to yourself means you know you won't be perfect so you have to leave room for error. So I began to give myself just that while still trying to make as few mistakes as possible.

I had a gym membership at Planet Fitness and I continued to use that gym membership as well as the great outdoors. There are many workouts you can look up for free on Pinterest, by following Instagram fitness influencers, and on YouTube. You can even search very targeted workouts for whatever area of your body you want to work out. I found workouts to do at the gym and I liked to switch it up at times by working out outside on pretty days. I found a change of scenery kept me from not getting too bored of the repetition of working out four to five times a week.

The more I worked out and stuck to my vegetarian diet, the more I witnessed my body letting go of weight. It was remarkable. Within a few days of being vegetarian I noticed my body losing fat a lot quicker than it did on any other diet. That is what encouraged me to dig deeper into my vegetarian diet. Since I let go of meat and seemed to be losing so much weight, I challenged myself to go vegan. My favorite cheat snack was ice cream and I loved cheese on many things, so I knew this would be tough. In the mornings, I was used to eating eggs too, so I had no idea how I was going to cut that out.

Just as I mentioned in chapter four, a paradigm shift, that is exactly what had happened next. I had a mental switch in the way I viewed eggs, cheese, and dairy by doing research from other vegans and nutritionists. Brace yourselves to read this...I started to look at eggs as a chicken's period because in actuality that is exactly what it is. Being a female, I know exactly what my eggs look like so why would I want to eat that from a chicken. Gross, I know. And I am sorry if I just killed your love for eggs. I continued to look up what eggs really are in nutrition and how they are farmed. The conditions that I witnessed the chickens being raised and bred in broke my heart so that was even more motivation for me to stop buying and eating eggs.

The paradigm shift to get me away from dairy came from me watching videos of how cows are treated in the factory farms and even the local farms. Local farms don't necessarily treat their cows inhumanely like the factory farms, but what female cows have to go through to produce milk was upsetting. To keep the cow producing milk, they basically have to continue being impregnated. The sad part is when they have their baby calf, the baby calf is immediately taken away from them. Call me crazy, but that breaks my heart, especially now as a breastfeeding mother. I can't imagine working so hard to produce so much milk only for another species to consume it. And it really breaks my heart to think about carrying my baby for nine months only to have him taken away from me right after birth. That is exactly what these cows go through, just to give us humans milk. All of that pain and torturing to a cow isn't worth it for me to have a glass of milk. This is nothing in comparison to what cows go through to be butchered for meat, but that is another story. Check out documentaries and movies for that insight.

The last thing I will share about cows and dairy is that I had to do my research and also feel my way through how dairy really affected me. What I mean by that is I had to listen intently to what my body was telling me. I had been drinking milk my entire life and consuming food products with dairy for so long that I didn't know what a clean body with no dairy felt like. When researching many forms of literature, they all said that dairy gave the body excess mucus. I had no idea what that meant; I simply thought more mucus must mean more snot in your nose, right?

I was proven wrong by my own body. I began to feel the changes within as I gave up dairy. Once I was dairy free for so long, anytime I would eat ice cream or something that had dairy in it, I would get the worst headache. I could feel the mucus build up in my head and I hated it. Knowing how it felt to be clean and free from this mucus that dairy gave me was a huge driving force in staying away from it. It was a new clarity that I appreciated my body for and I felt bad for treating my body so wrong before. When you know better you do better right?

Once I was able to transition from being vegetarian to vegan, I felt great! I had never felt better. Before my trip to Vegas, I challenged myself even more to go "raw vegan." Everything that I had to eat had to be in its natural state like fresh fruit, vegetables, nuts, etc. I was able to maintain this raw vegan diet for a little over a week, as it was harder to sustain on our trip to Las Vegas. I did try to stick to the raw vegan as much as possible, except one of the restaurants we ate at had a cooked butternut squash soup.

When I came home from Las Vegas, I went back to my regular vegan diet no problem. Yet, for some reason I was able to eat an entire watermelon by myself and I couldn't put the jar of pickles down. I also noticed a change in my attitude while I was at work. When I arrived at Planet Fitness for an afternoon workout on May 14, 2018 I realized I had on sandals. How the heck was I supposed to workout in open-toe sandals? It was at that moment I realized I was eating way more than normal, my attitude had changed, my memory was not on point, and not to mention my nails were growing at the rate of a monster. You are catching my drift, right? Could I be pregnant?

Luckily there was a Dollar Store next to Planet Fitness so I walked to the store, bought one pregnancy test stick, peed on it, and sure enough. There was a plus sign in no time and it hit me. I had way too much fun in Vegas and now I am pregnant. Honestly, my first emotion was disappointment that I was finally at the fittest point in my life and I popped up pregnant. I started to pray about it, talked it over with my fiance at the time (now hubby), and came to terms with it. I started to view it for what it truly was, a blessing by all means!

I was gung-ho for staying vegan throughout my pregnancy. I just knew I was going to be able to do it. But as the weeks progressed and I was on the road more and more, I realized it was getting harder to sustain my vegan diet while traveling so much. Prior to being pregnant when I would travel, if I couldn't find a vegan option to eat in Southern Louisiana, I would juice, drink water, or simply fast. I understood that missing a meal is not an option while carrying and growing a child. That was when I realized it wasn't about me anymore so I started making exceptions and eating meat here and there.

Being pregnant and adjusting my diet was not the hard part. The season of motherhood that really broke my vegan ways was breastfeeding. I was even hungrier breastfeeding than I was when I was pregnant. There were days when I would nurse and try to eat vegan, but because it contained so many green veggies, fiber, and beans, the milk I produced gave my infant gas. I had to do what was best for him, so I ate what my mom cooked for me because she wanted to help out as much as she could. And if you know my mom, she isn't much of a cook so her meal options were pretty limited. That meant I ate tuna casserole, meatloaf and veggies, and eggs because that is what my mom prepared for me. I was grateful for the food and that I had her help, but it was a sacrifice I had to make in my vegan ways to continue breastfeeding my son.

When my little one was a year old, I started to go back to my vegan habits as his stomach was not as sensitive as it was when he was a newborn. At this time, with him being older, I had more time on my hands too, so prepping my own vegan meals became easier. I still continued to breastfeed my little man, but he didn't need as much as he did when he was hitting those major milestones during the infancy stage. Currently, my little one is fifteen months and I stick to a primarily vegan diet while still nursing him every now and then.

One major lesson I have recently learned is that our immune systems in our bodies all start with gut health. Since having my son, I have had the flu and strep throat all within fourteen months. However, when I was vegan, and even vegetarian, I never got sick once in over two years. Why was my immune system so strong then, but weakened as I began to eat meat? It is because it all starts in your gut.

The biological term is Gastrointestinal Microbiota, and that is your gut flora. I am no medical doctor, scientist, or even nutritionist (yet), so when it comes to understanding how the body works, I like to keep it simple! I keep it simple by knowing my body and whether or not I am adding good bacteria or bad. I have learned over time that when I am eating rice and gravy, gumbo, jambalaya, or lots of meat, I get sick easier. On the opposite spectrum, when I am eating fruits and veggies that aid in boosting my immune system, it is alot harder for me to get sick. I don't know about you, but I love keeping my body healthy and happy to fight off germs and viruses, so that is another huge reason I stick to my vegan diet. Compromising my health by eating whatever is available may be the cheaper and easier thing to do, especially in social situations; yet, it is most definitely not worth it to me when I end up sick as a dog later on because I didn't take care of my gut.

In a nutshell, that is my journey from eating meat, to going vegetarian, to vegan, to back to my carnivorous ways, back to what I am now. Through it all, I have learned to not let it define me. My eating preferences are simply decisions that I make and not necessarily who I am. I used to be a stickler and define myself as a vegan. I don't like to do that anymore because I am so much more than just what I eat and what I believe in. I also feel that by categorizing myself as "a vegan" it makes me unrelatable to those who aren't, but still want to try to eat better.

One thing vegans, vegetarians, and other people out there who eat better for a cleaner world and a better version of themselves need to do is encourage and uplift one another. We shouldn't put each other down because of our differences. When I lived in Atlanta and made lots of vegan friends, they were very judgemental. The reason some vegans can be so tough to non-vegans, myself included, is because we believe in the cause so much! We believe in saving our environment, we believe in saving the animals, and most importantly we believe in saving ourselves and living as optimally as possible. I get why vegans can sometimes come off very hard and judgemental, but I encourage us all to do some reflection, both on ourselves as well as on other people's lives, to come to a more understanding standpoint versus a critiquing one. Maybe someone can't eat as clean as you'd like them to for medical reasons. Maybe someone can't eat as many fruits and vegetables as you'd like them to because of where they live. What matters is that they are trying to do better, not perfectionism remember?

I am excited for you to go on a healthier journey and incorporate some of the vegan habits I have shared with you. Be sure to follow me on social media for inspiration and to stay tuned and watch how the journey continues. I am now aiming for an even cleaner pregnancy than my first, challenging myself to fully stick to my vegan diet, even with a tiny human growing inside of me. I know it is possible as I have seen many healthy pregnancies done before by other vegan eaters, so that is a personal goal I have set for myself in the future. Once you follow me on social media, I will be more than happy to do the same for you as our betterment journey continues!

More Books from This Author

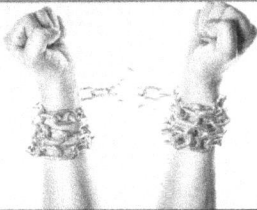

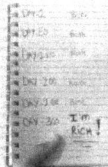

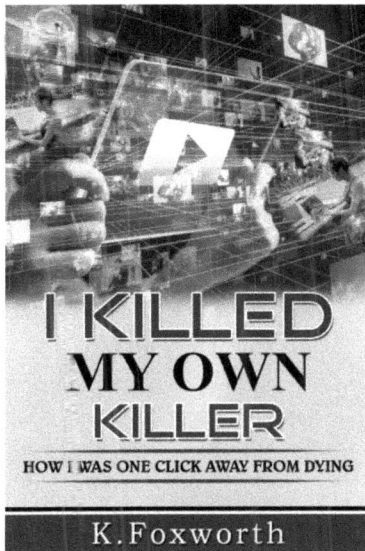

(

About the Author

I had graduated Louisiana State University in 2016 and had always believed in entrepreneurship. I told myself as I received my diploma, "This is a pretty diploma, but I hope I never have to use it unless it is working for my own business."

At that time, I did not know what I really wanted to do, but I knew I wanted it to do three things for me.

1. Create a life that I (and God) had complete control over. I didn't want a boss telling me how much money I could make, when to take my lunch break, or when I could have time off of work.

2. I wanted freedom and flexibility to spend everyday where I wanted and with whom I wanted. I wanted to be with my husband everyday if I chose to because he was indeed my best friend. I wanted to hang out with my

puppies (later on kids) by the pool at one in the afternoon just because I could. And I wanted to get up and go be with my family for days because I had the time and money to do it.

3. Most importantly I wanted what I did to bring me closer to my maker everyday. I knew the only way I could make that happen was by impacting a lot of people.

So that is what I chose to do. I did not know how I was going to do it. I just knew I wasn't going to settle for anything less.

In making this decision, my family started this pattern of thinking I was crazy. How was I going to graduate college and not work a job? I must be out of my mind, right?

Then I started to piece all the puzzles of my life together from my darkest moments of attempted suicide to my brightest moments of graduating and getting engaged.

Everything we go through in life has a reason. One of my fondest memories is when I would pass KFC with my Uncle P. He would say, "KFC doesn't mean Kentucky Fried Chicken. It means Katelyn's Freaking Crazy!" I would laugh so hard every time he'd say that to me.

Growing up, I knew he was joking and that always made me laugh. But when I went vegan all I could think of was, "Damn! Katelyn is *freakin' crazy!* Once again..." That is what everyone in Louisiana would tell me as I gave up more and more meat.

That was a breaking point for me as I sought out my own independence, relying only on God and myself, that I was not only going to use this *crazy* dietary change to impact me, but I wanted it to affect others.

But how? Then I made an even crazier move! I left little Louisiana for the big and almighty Atlanta! That is when everyone from my hometown really thought **"Katelyn's freakin' crazy!"** I used this familiar saying in my life as a huge motivation to make the impossible possible!

As my life progressed, I realized my family might be right. I just may be crazy because my choices don't always follow "the norm" or what most people would do. After going vegan, moving to Atlanta, and then getting pregnant in Vegas, I decided I wanted to have my baby naturally. By naturally, I do mean vaginally and with *no* epidural! That blew the socks off of a lot of my family's minds because they are huge fans of using medicines to heal your body or take the pain away. But if you haven't gotten the point by now, I like to do things the natural way. Once again, OMG KFC, Katelyn is Freaking Crazy!

Mission accomplished! On January 4, 2019, I delivered my baby boy all natural after being induced with no medication. That is why my husband and I joke that my alter-ego is indeed KFV: Katelyn's Freakin Vegan. Even though I am not full-on vegan, we like to say that KFV lives inside of me and she always will.

I hope you've enjoyed the crazy KFV experience as you embark on your own journey. So when you are about to do something crazy like order a salad when all of your friends are getting burgers and beer to watch the game think, "OMG KFV! If she could do it, so could I!" I promise you won't regret it.

Daily Affirmations Guideline Copies

Fill in this positive affirmation below for you to read to yourself DAILY!

I, _____ am ready for a great day and it all starts with my health and attitude! I will choose to eat healthier foods today such as:

_____

_____

(list whatever meals you have prepped, healthy foods you have at home and at work)

I know that the foods I choose to eat will have an impact on how I feel, how I look on the outside, and how I see myself. I want to feel

_____

(what do you want to change emotionally? Ex: to feel happier at the end of the day, more vibrant when you wake up, more energy when with your family, etc.)

I will look like

_____

on the outside. *(Specific weight loss goal, physical feature, or personal example. Ex: to look like Gina Rodriguez, to lose my love handles, or decrease my back fat, to lose 5 lbs. in the next 2 weeks)*

I will see myeslf as

_____

_____

(This can be how you see yourself emotionally and physically. How do you want to see yourself that you don't see yourself as now. Make sure it is super positive and uplifting and repeat it in your head as your day goes on. Examples: a strong and healthy-eating warrior wife ready to conquer my career, a loving and fit mother who sets a great example for her kids while exercising and taking care of herself daily, a busy yet healthy student with strong muscles and sharp brain.)

Fill in this positive affirmation below for you to read to yourself DAILY!

I, _____ am ready for a great day and it all starts with my health and attitude! I will choose to eat healthier foods today such as:

_____

_____

(list whatever meals you have prepped, healthy foods you have at home and at work)

I know that the foods I choose to eat will have an impact on how I feel, how I look on the outside, and how I see myself. I want to feel

_____

(what do you want to change emotionally? Ex: to feel happier at the end of the day, more vibrant when you wake up, more energy when with your family, etc.)

I will look like

_____

on the outside. (*Specific weight loss goal, physical feature, or personal example. Ex: to look like Gina Rodriguez, to lose my love handles, or decrease my back fat, to lose 5 lbs. in the next 2 weeks*)

I will see myeslf as

_____

(This can be how you see yourself emotionally and physically. How do you want to see yourself that you don't see yourself as now Make sure it is super positive and uplifting and repeat it in your head as your day goes on. Examples: a strong and healthy-eating warrior wife ready to conquer my career, a loving and fit mother who sets a great example for her kids while exercising and taking care of herself daily, a busy yet healthy student with strong muscles and sharp brain.)

Fill in this positive affirmation below for you to read to yourself DAILY!

I, _____ am ready for a great day and it all starts with my health and attitude! I will choose to eat healthier foods today such as:

_____

_____

(list whatever meals you have prepped, healthy foods you have at home and at work)

I know that the foods I choose to eat will have an impact on how I feel, how I look on the outside, and how I see myself. I want to feel

_____

(what do you want to change emotionally? Ex: to feel happier at the end of the day, more vibrant when you wake up, more energy when with your family, etc.)

I will look like

_____

on the outside. *(Specific weight loss goal, physical feature, or personal example. Ex: to look like Gina Rodriguez, to lose my love handles, or decrease my back fat, to lose 5 lbs. in the next 2 weeks)*

I will see myeslf as

_____

_____

(This can be how you see yourself emotionally and physically. How do you want to see yourself that you don't see yourself as now Make sure it is super positive and uplifting and repeat it in your head as your day goes on. Examples: a strong and healthy-eating warrior wife ready to conquer my career, a loving and fit mother who sets a great example for her kids while exercising and taking care of herself daily, a busy yet healthy student with strong muscles and sharp brain.)

Fill in this positive affirmation below for you to read to yourself DAILY!

I, _____ am ready for a great day and it all starts with my health and attitude! I will choose to eat healthier foods today such as:

_____

_____

(list whatever meals you have prepped, healthy foods you have at home and at work)

I know that the foods I choose to eat will have an impact on how I feel, how I look on the outside, and how I see myself. I want to feel

_____

(what do you want to change emotionally? Ex: to feel happier at the end of the day, more vibrant when you wake up, more energy when with your family, etc.)

I will look like

_____

on the outside. *(Specific weight loss goal, physical feature, or personal example. Ex: to look like Gina Rodriguez, to lose my love handles, or decrease my back fat, to lose 5 lbs. in the next 2 weeks)*

I will see myeslf as

_____

(This can be how you see yourself emotionally and physically. How do you want to see yourself that you don't see yourself as now Make sure it is super positive and uplifting and repeat it in your head as your day goes on. Examples: a strong and healthy-eating warrior wife ready to conquer my career, a loving and fit mother who sets a great example for her kids while exercising and taking care of herself daily, a busy yet healthy student with strong muscles and sharp brain.)

Fill in this positive affirmation below for you to read to yourself DAILY!

I, _____ am ready for a great day and it all starts with my health and attitude! I will choose to eat healthier foods today such as:

_____

_____

(list whatever meals you have prepped, healthy foods you have at home and at work)

I know that the foods I choose to eat will have an impact on how I feel, how I look on the outside, and how I see myself. I want to feel

_____

(what do you want to change emotionally? Ex: to feel happier at the end of the day, more vibrant when you wake up, more energy when with your family, etc.)

I will look like

_____

on the outside. *(Specific weight loss goal, physical feature, or personal example. Ex: to look like Gina Rodriguez, to lose my love handles, or decrease my back fat, to lose 5 lbs. in the next 2 weeks)*

I will see myeslf as

_____

_____

(This can be how you see yourself emotionally and physically. How do you want to see yourself that you don't see yourself as now Make sure it is super positive and uplifting and repeat it in your head as your day goes on. Examples: a strong and healthy-eating warrior wife ready to conquer my career, a loving and fit mother who sets a great example for her kids while exercising and taking care of herself daily, a busy yet healthy student with strong muscles and sharp brain.)

Fill in this positive affirmation below for you to read to yourself DAILY!

I, _____ am ready for a great day and it all starts with my health and attitude! I will choose to eat healthier foods today such as:

_____

_____

(list whatever meals you have prepped, healthy foods you have at home and at work)

I know that the foods I choose to eat will have an impact on how I feel, how I look on the outside, and how I see myself. I want to feel

_____

(what do you want to change emotionally? Ex: to feel happier at the end of the day, more vibrant when you wake up, more energy when with your family, etc.)

I will look like

_____

on the outside. *(Specific weight loss goal, physical feature, or personal example. Ex: to look like Gina Rodriguez, to lose my love handles, or decrease my back fat, to lose 5 lbs. in the next 2 weeks)*

I will see myeslf as

_____

(This can be how you see yourself emotionally and physically. How do you want to see yourself that you don't see yourself as now Make sure it is super positive and uplifting and repeat it in your head as your day goes on. Examples: a strong and healthy-eating warrior wife ready to conquer my career, a loving and fit mother who sets a great example for her kids while exercising and taking care of herself daily, a busy yet healthy student with strong muscles and sharp brain.)

Fill in this positive affirmation below for you to read to yourself DAILY!

I, _____ am ready for a great day and it all starts with my health and attitude! I will choose to eat healthier foods today such as:

_____

_____

(list whatever meals you have prepped, healthy foods you have at home and at work)

I know that the foods I choose to eat will have an impact on how I feel, how I look on the outside, and how I see myself. I want to feel

_____

(what do you want to change emotionally? Ex: to feel happier at the end of the day, more vibrant when you wake up, more energy when with your family, etc.)

I will look like

_____

on the outside. (*Specific weight loss goal, physical feature, or personal example. Ex: to look like Gina Rodriguez, to lose my love handles, or decrease my back fat, to lose 5 lbs. in the next 2 weeks*)

I will see myeslf as

_____

(This can be how you see yourself emotionally and physically. How do you want to see yourself that you don't see yourself as now Make sure it is super positive and uplifting and repeat it in your head as your day goes on. Examples: a strong and healthy-eating warrior wife ready to conquer my career, a loving and fit mother who sets a great example for her kids while exercising and taking care of herself daily, a busy yet healthy student with strong muscles and sharp brain.)